Mario Zaidenberg

The path to Malaria elimination in Argentina

AF155367

Mario Zaidenberg

The path to Malaria elimination in Argentina

LAP LAMBERT Academic Publishing

Publisher:
LAP LAMBERT Academic Publishing
is a trademark of
Dodo Books Indian Ocean Ltd. and OmniScriptum S.R.L publishing group

120 High Road, East Finchley, London, N2 9ED, United Kingdom
Str. Armeneasca 28/1, office 1, Chisinau MD-2012, Republic of Moldova, Europe
Managing Directors: Ieva Konstantinova, Victoria Ursu
info@omniscriptum.com

Printed at: see last page
ISBN: 978-3-659-80500-4

THE PATH TO MALARIA ELIMINATION IN ARGENTINA

The long road of evolution of malaria in Argentina since the last decade of the nineteenth century to the present

Mario Zaidenberg
MsC Epidemiology

INDEX

1. INTRODUCTION

The history of malaria in Argentina encompasses an extended period of over a hundred years of evolution since the late 19th century to the present. Over these years, there were different experiences, guidelines, methods and, primarily, protagonists of this lengthy process as well as different scenarios that witnessed the attack of a disease that gave no break to the long-suffering inhabitants. This long period has been arbitrarily divided into four phases, each characterized by particular features.

The **First phase** encompassed the period between 1891 and 1939, and was characterized by prevailing environmental engineering works for malaria control. The endemic disease jeopardized more than eight provinces; thousands of people suffered from the impact of a disease that weakened the already diminished forces of suffering people in the central and northern part of the country. At this phase efforts were focused on reducing the impact of the disease using the Italian sanitary engineering method. This method aimed at reducing or avoiding the influence of water sources in the formation of anopheles mosquito breeding sites by constructing embankments and landfills, evacuating flooded areas or wetlands, straightening streambeds, etc., and distributing quinine in the endemic area.

Structural poverty of those years was a daily presence accompanying the suffering of the local population, as evidenced by the testimony of qualified witnesses, (1), "... life is also very sad in the "ranchos" (local name for small and poor farmhouses). There vegetate these poor families, almost everyone provided with nothing more than one dark, narrow room, deprived of all hygiene and comfort conditions, exposed to severe weather, in the company of dogs, cats, etc., that is, living with them and, in a word, reduced to the most miserable conditions..."

In this particularly difficult environment, this phase showed no evident improvements in the occurrence of cases and was characterized by the criticisms by local researchers who claimed that the european methods used were not suitable for the local malaria vectors, which showed different habits. Thus, the **Second phase** begins in a scenario of a very important endemic disease that was affecting the health of thousands of people, and limited urban and/or suburban developments in the most important towns of that time, which intended to prevent or reduce the risk of malaria infection. This phase is marked by the appearance of a new insecticide, **D**ichloro **D**iphenyl **T**richloroethane or DDT, which has a determining impact on the endemic disease, causing the most significant reduction known in the endemic area until then, and the deployment of work teams in charge of systematic spraying during a limited period but that marked the epidemiological malaria scenario in Argentina forever.

At the **Third phase, 1950 - 2008**, previous achievements were gradually consolidated: the malaria transmission area was reduced and a method for epidemiological surveillance was established, which still survives to date, with little modifications. Field work at this phase was conditioned by epidemiological variations of this and other vector-borne diseases, such as dengue and Chagas disease. The same technical personnel were responsible for the respective activities, according to the assigned priorities, and since 1998 in particular, with the advent of dengue in Argentina, they were subject to epidemic variants of the disease.

The **Forth phase**: at this contemporary phase, 2009 - 2015, the epidemiological situation in the country is stratified according to an updated evaluation; in addition, appropriate evolution control indicators are achieved, which are the basis for claiming that indigenous transmission of malaria in the country has stopped or been eliminated.

Thus, this is a brief account of the four stages that marked out the route towards the elimination of malaria in Argentina and that we intend to describe in the following pages.

2. FIRST PHASE
1891 – 1939

The history of malaria control in Argentina refers the late 19th century, in 1886 as a significant milestone, when Dr. Eliseo Canton submitted his thesis to obtain the degree of medical doctor in the University of Buenos Aires: "Study of Malaria in the province of Tucuman". Five years later he published a basic work: "Malaria and medical geography in Argentina". Dr. Canton observed malaria as a result of the unhealthy environment landscapes that generate germs of malaria. He described the health conditions of various parts of the northwestern region, showing the vast magnitude and the local variation in malaria problem. He advocated for malaria control not only for its health benefits, but also for the potential economic benefits that would be derived from agriculture, industry and local governments. Dr. Canton believed that the most efficient and long-lasting means of malaria control were the elimination of the sources of infection, which meant the disinfection of unhealthy landscapes through drainage, cultivation, tree planting, and other rational and productive land uses, (2).

Since the beginning of 1900, control activities were basically distributed in two areas: environmental, including advising enterprises which due to their nature could create favorable conditions for the breeding of the vector, such as railways, roads, dams and projects on streams; and health care, involving the distribution and supply of quinine to accessible populations in urban and suburban areas.

An example of this concept is a reference to Dr Antenor Alvarez, (3), who managed the control of malaria epidemic in Santiago del Estero between 1900 and 1903. "The completion of the dam against river floods led to the diversion of the water flow of the branch passing in front of the city. Once the flow of this branch was stopped, a focus with all malarial conditions was formed, with malaria bursting in the surrounding area, which remained localized for a short time, and later invaded the entire city and surrounding departments with alarming characteristics in its intensity and spread. The urban population amounted to 11409 inhabitants, of which 8243 people became ill with malaria; infection rate of 72.2%. The recommendations to manage the situation were: "Avoid draining in the marsh focus..., remove the mouth-intakes from ditches..., drain the marsh focus, dry and proceed to the malarious area earthworks..., planting hundreds of eucalyptus in the vicinity of the focus...". This, along with quinine administration, helped to control the epidemic in August 1903.

The cited paragraph clearly illustrates the prevailing concept in the country regarding the approach to malaria problem; at the same time, through the implemented actions the etiologic role of mosquitoes in the genesis of the malaria problem is demonstrated.

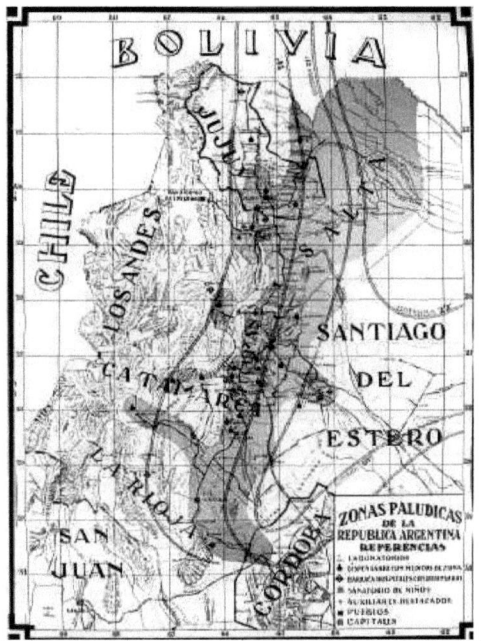

Figure N° 1. Map of Malarious Zones from Nicolás Lozano. Profilaxis del Paludismo, (Buenos Aires, La Semana Médica, 1909). Courtesy of the National University of Mar del Plata, Argentina.

In this epidemic the prevalent vector, *Anopheles pseudopunctipennis* (4) had been already identified. However, given the medical concepts of that time, the identification of the vector was not specifically translated into the control strategy of the endemic, which continued with the methodology based on environmental engineering works. Between 1904 and 1911, several researchers in Argentina, such as doctors Felix Garzón

Maceda, Juan Carlos Delfino, Carlos M. Albarracin, Carlos Canavesio, Miguel A. Figueroa, Antonio Filardi, Pedro J. Garcia, Hector Quintana, William Ruzzo and Carlos Vera, published articles on etiology, transmission, environment, clinical forms, malaria treatment, etc., which contributed to the characterization of malaria in the country, (5).

In October 1911, the law of defense against malaria (Act N° 5195) was regulated; this law established the legal, administrative and technical bases for malaria control, (6). It provided in legal, administrative and technical terms the guidelines to follow in line with the scientific knowledge of that time. It established among other aspects: "... It is declared mandatory in national jurisdiction to report any cases of malaria that may occur, to the nearest local authority, so that the appropriate medical care is provided." It indicated the people responsible for law enforcement, established fines, and, more importantly, enabled the creation of the Malaria Service, under the direction of the National Department of Health, (NHD) with authority to work in the provinces affected by the disease, and indicated that "...Governments of the provinces, must recognize the immediate intervention of the National Hygiene Department and the centralization of leading action of the malaria control campaign."

In the body of the law there was a communication from the Chair of the Department of Hygiene addressed to the Honorable Advisory Council, which established the strategy to be followed: "... showing two fundamental prophylactic methods or systems: one destined to act on people (internal prophylaxis) by the continued administration of quinine; another one (external prophylaxis), which can be further divided into two branches: one concerning the fight against mosquitoes and their larvae (direct measures) and the other (indirect measures) comprising the drainage of lands susceptible to facilitate the development of these insects, recognized as accurate and obligate vectors of the malaria parasites."

Article 21 established that "those suffering from malaria, whose existence is known in any form" should receive free medical assistance and health treatment in the provinces and territories..." The article also urged the NHD to spread the knowledge regarding protection against malaria among the population." using all the available means.

In the same year, Guillermo Patterson, in Jujuy, stated that the most important epidemiological vector of malaria in northwestern Argentina was *Anopheles pseudopunctipennis* (7). G. Patterson was an English doctor who had an outstanding performance in various activities such as malaria, leishmaniasis and Chagas in northwestern Argentina. He lived in the province of Jujuy and developed his professional work in San Pedro, Ledesma and Santa Bárbara departments of that province, where he was appointed delegate of the National Department of Hygiene by Malbrán.

Dr. Paterson made an interesting account of the disease in the region. "The history of malaria in the region dates back to about 35 years ago, in 1876, when the first attempts were made to grow coffee and sugar cane in the initial plantations of the towns San Pedro, Ledesma and Calilegua, in the province of Jujuy. The story told by those who cleared the lands narrates the extraordinary spread of malaria at that time. Neither the farm workers nor the company employees could escape from it; fevers were serious and persistent. Thus, the "chucho" (popular concept of malaria disease and / or chills) of San Pedro acquired the same name as that of the Frontier's "chucho" where it occurred in a severe form". Once the larva breeding sites were detected, predominantly along San Pedro Stream and the railroad, the algae that served as food for the mosquito larvae was eliminated using tar. Repeated interventions gave a transient success, which systematically led to a renewed disease attack, which generated a number of questions and so many frustrations. The efforts made, even those that originated a justified optimism, were offset by the spread of mosquito and the increase of the disease", (8).

Malarial available indicators were a proof of the vulnerability of populations in the north of the country, including the provinces of Salta, Tucuman, La Rioja and Catamarca.

Table N° 1. Malaria morbidity in endemic provinces of Argentina, 1912-1915

YEARS	TUCUMAN	SALTA	JUJUY	CATAMARCA	LA RIOJA	TOTAL
1912	19909	19790	8833	5420	1372	55324
1913	62145	39410	13505	10475	3052	128587
1914	96170	44977	14914	14598	3966	174625
1915	84209	43119	18615	13154	3728	162825
TOTAL 12-15	262433	147296	55867	43647	12118	521361
ANNUAL AV.	65608	36824	13967	10912	3030	130340

Source: Jose Penna and Antonio Barbieri, Malaria and its prophylaxis in Argentina (Buenos Aires: DNH, 1916), 68-69.

From 1915 to 1935 antimalaria interventions became widely known in the country. Regional offices were set up in the provinces, one of which was in Jujuy. The action was focused on two areas: the environmental area, with sanitation projects consisting of hydraulic engineering works -drainage and landfills-, and human health area, for which dispensaries were created for distributing quinine among people exposed to the disease.

In 1925, at the request of Dr. Gregorio Araoz Alfaro, the Rockefeller Foundation was invited to work in the country. Work was conducted in Ledesma and La Esperanza sugar mills, in Tucuman and Jujuy. The Foundation provided funds and an environmental engineer for performing slopes, drains, ditches and other adaptations of the environment in subtropical areas of the plantations. Cooperative work was conducted for four years but failed to achieve the expected results. The issue came to the Chamber of Deputies. There, the deputy Gimenez presented a report about the situation in the northwestern region. Calling it "...The endemic disease that plagues large regions, ruining the coefficient of the individual energies, especially in the working mass" he addressed the issue of options to overcome such difficult problem, and of all the available ones, he proposed applying all the techniques known until then. He stated that all works were carried out in populated localities of endemic areas in northern Argentina, "but the vast expanse of fields, villages and scattered rural hamlets, where high morbidity persists, remains unattended, and shows how difficult it is to fight because of unsanitary housing, poverty and long distances, and the results are so disproportionate compared to the expenses it requires. Improving this requires a technical organization with central control and direction of the National Department of Health, since no uniform plan has been conceived", (5,8).

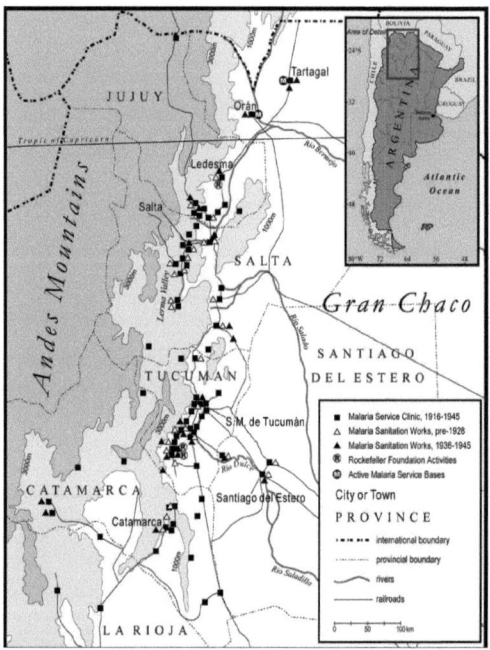

Figure N°. 2. Map of the northwestern region of Argentina, with malaria control campaign clinics and sanitation project works of the National Hygiene Department, (DNH), activities of the Rockefeller Foundation and current malaria service bases. Other cartographic details (railways, borders) are approximately from 1930. Sources: Barbieri 1928; General Directorate of Malaria 1938-1946; DNH 1920; DNH 1938; Penna and Barbieri 1916; geographic information provided by the Geographical Survey Institute, National University of Tucuman.
Eric Carter, Paludismo, Sociedad y Medio ambiente en el Noroeste argentino a principios del siglo Veinte. pp 27., Grinnell College, Iowa, USA.

Descriptions of entomological aspects agreed that in three endemic provinces, Salta, Jujuy and Tucuman, the findings very frequently reported the presence of *An. pseudopunctipennis*, which was found in large numbers, primarily in thatched-roof huts ("quincha") and bathrooms as preferred resting sites and in dark sites, often in stables in large quantities. *"In general we can say that: the darker and dirtier, and the less aired rooms, the more preferred are by anopheles"* (9). Other specimens mentioned were *An argyritarsis, albitarsis*. In Salta, the most abundant was *An argyritarsis*, followed by *An tarsimaculata, An pseudopunctipennis* and *An albitarsis*, with *An pseudopunctipennis* being the one most frequently found in the rooms.

The entomological material collected in the provinces of Chaco and Formosa during October included: *An albitarsis* and several culicids. These researchers stressed the social conditions of the local population, "Noting that malaria is primarily a disease of poverty and the poorest..., and they remember the vicious circle between pauperism and alcoholism that will determine a state of lower resistance, of indolence and fatalism which can lead to future degeneration of those populations", (ibid).

regard to the fight against malaria, they described how difficult the task was and they concluded that it was imperative that all people should cooperate with the State authorities and medical doctors; that education should begin at school with good health education and in people's homes; they recommended strengthening the systematic treatment with quinine and, for adult anopheles, fumigations with an alcohol solution of pyrethrum using sprayers available in the northern provinces. They insisted that the best means of protection against mosquito bites was always a properly implemented mosquito net during the night and house protection by covering doors and windows with fine-wire netting. Regarding anopheles breeding sites, they recommended the systematic elimination of small areas of standing water and pools near the houses, cleaning and channeling all large ponds, conducting drainage and removing vegetation that favors larval development, regulation and cleaning of the margins of streams and rivers; when the ponds, ditches and pools could not be removed or channeled, petroleum, saprol larvicide or any other larvicidal should be poured over the water surface at a rate of 20-30 cm^3 per square meter every two months, during the season of larval development.

Shannon EC, Davis NC and E. del Ponte, (12), characterized *An pseudopunctipennis* mainly as a highland species, which prefers to breed in the waters of streams and springs, and in ponds that are formed on their margins. There are vast semi-arid plains to the east and southeast that pose insurmountable barriers to expansion. According to the knowledge of that time, the species was confined to the western or Andean region (and adjacent lowlands), west of the low central area that obviously serves as a barrier to expansion. They also noted that the species was more abundant at the end of the rainy season. Among other findings, they described entomological aspects for the littoral area, along the Bermejo, Parana and Paraguay rivers, comprising the riparian areas of these rivers in the provinces of Corrientes, Santa Fe, Chaco, Formosa and Misiones. They assumed that *An pseudopunctipennis* was not the problem in the area, but that vectors responsible for the transmission might belong to the *Nysshorynchus* (*albitarsis, argyritarsis* and *tarsimaculatus*) group.

From 1916 to 1935, malaria control received a significant boost from the European schools of malariology, particularly by the Italian one, mainly based on environmental sanitation works. Major anti-malaria engineering works were also undertaken, with canalizations, drainage and landfills, and distribution of quinine in rural areas was increased; this period was described as "drainage and quinine", (5). However, epidemiological indicators showed an endemic stabilization in affected areas without effective improvement.

Dr. Antonio Barbieri, head of the Malaria sector, publishes the advances made in control in the last 10 years, and "says that thanks to a system that followed the example of most experimented countries, malaria control was a success, as well as sanitation combined with quininization, which had reduced disease incidence in the northwest, especially in large cities. (11).

Barbieri was the head of the National Department of Health (DNH) in 1933 and continued his general distribution policy of combined quinine, and when financially possible, with sanitation interventions, but no original research about the disease was conducted during that time.

Sanitation had been originated in the era of miasma; in Argentina it was implemented during the epidemic of Santiago del Estero; it was formalized with the Law 5195 and the work done by the Malaria program, and validated by the Italian experience.

In the last years of this period, however, some professionals were not satisfied with the evolution of the endemic until those years, and based on different experiences, determined relevant features of the bionomics of local anopheles, in particular with the behavior related to the conditioning microenvironment. Among these professionals were the medical doctors Guillermo Paterson, Carlos Alvarado, Juana Petrocchi and Alois Bachmann, who established fundamental works in the evolution of malaria control in Argentina, (7,13,14,15).

Accordingly, there was a key meeting in 1934, the Ninth Pan American Sanitary Conference, held in Buenos Aires, in which the president of the DNH at that time, Dr. Miguel Sussini, responsible for control actions, presents the case against environmental sanitation and the need for a new approach, (13,16). At this key meeting, Sussini questioned the old methods, showing their false analogies, reconsidered the oldest scientific evidence and offered an alternative model: "foci patrol" or "foci police", which suited the northwestern geographic and epidemiological conditions. "With this approach," said Sussini, "Regional Director of Jujuy, Dr. Carlos Alberto Alvarado, began a series of observations that sought to fill the remaining gaps in the knowledge of the habits of *An pseudopunctipennis*; especially concerning the behavior of this species during non-reproductive periods and their preferred breeding conditions, also seeking to establish the circumstances that link, associate or dissociate the various anopheline species and their relationships with their respective environments..."; in his presentation, Sussini also cited the work of scientists at the Rockefeller Foundation, Davis, Rickard and Raymond Shannon as a crucial improvement in the understanding of *pseudopunctipennis*, particularly in three areas: host preference, flight range and preferred breeding sites. These researchers confirmed an important anthropophilic behavior of *An. pseudopunctipennis* compared with other anopheles, thereby confirming the findings of Paterson de 1911, (7).

The article "Las fiebres palúdicas en Jujuy" (Malarial fevers in Jujuy), written by Guillermo Paterson, and published in 1911, (7), was critical for the ending of the controversy between the protagonists of the substantial difference in health strategy of Esperanza, sugar mill in San Pedro, Jujuy, which struggled against malaria endemic from 1894 to 1943. Paterson, one of the key members of the regional pathologist network in the northwest, was an English doctor who supervised the clinical area. During his stay there, already in 1899, he dedicated to investigate the local epidemiology of malaria and examined the habits of local mosquitoes. In his publication in 1911, Paterson set two points that eventually came to be of great importance. First, he determined that *An* p*seudopunctipennis* was the most outstanding species in the areas of Jujuy and Salta, where malaria was common.

The presence of this species was almost invariably associated with the disease, unlike the presence of other species, such as *Anopheles argyritarsis*.

The dominant presence of *An. pseudopunctipennis* in domestic environments led Paterson to argue that it was "virtually the only species that acts as a spreading agent for malaria" in the area, (4).

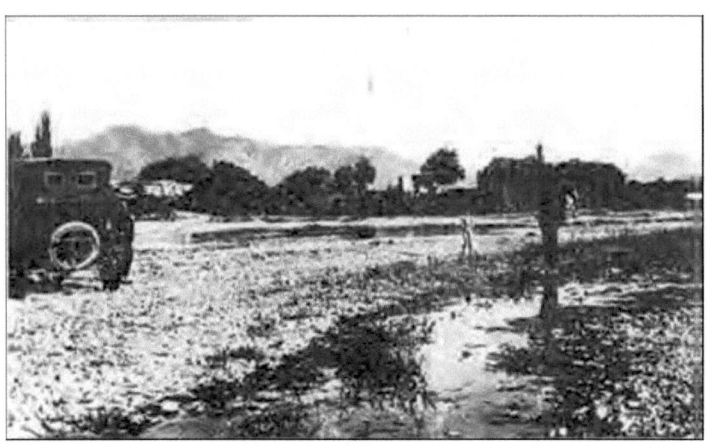

Photo N° 1. *An pseudopunctipennis* larval breeding sites in Arias River, Salta, 1926, (12)

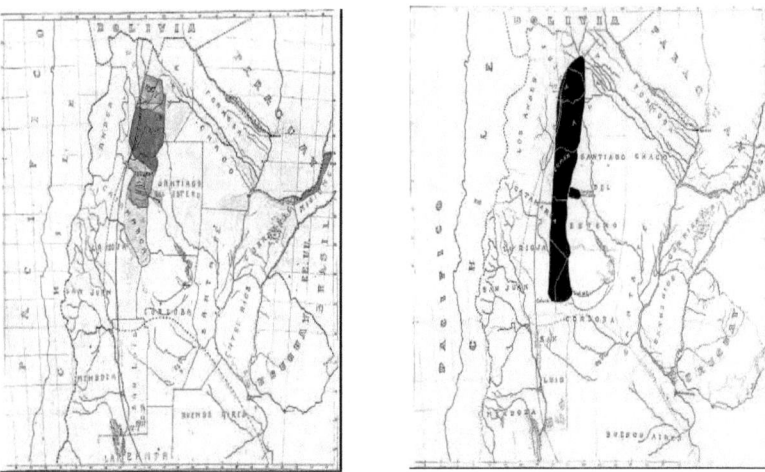

Figures N°. 3 and 4. Distribution of Malaria and *An pseudopunctipennis* in Argentina, 1927, (12).

Secondly, according to numerous observations Paterson characterized a typical *An pseudopunctipennis* breeding area as breeding sites found in clear waters, and preferably in those containing certain types of multicellular algae, associated with *Spirogyra*, that were the favorite food of the *An pseudopunctipennis* larvae. In a table, Paterson indicated the main breeding sites –springs, streams and wells–, which prevailed, whereas marshes were rarely mentioned.

In the cited work of Shannon, Davis and del Ponte,(12), they emphasized the overlap of the most affected areas by the disease with *An. pseudopunctipennis* distribution area, and concluded that this species is not found in places where malaria is nonexistent or unimportant (e.g., Corrientes and Chaco).

Later they explored how malaria was transmitted in northeastern Argentina and proposed two possibilities: 1) as an invasion by *An pseudopunctipennis* from Bermejo River and 2) a more likely scenario that they assumed as an extension of Alto Paraná mediated by other anopheles.

Regarding *An pseudopunctipennis*, they described it mainly as a species from mountain areas and, secondly, that their favorite breeding sites would be water flows, springs and associated pools.

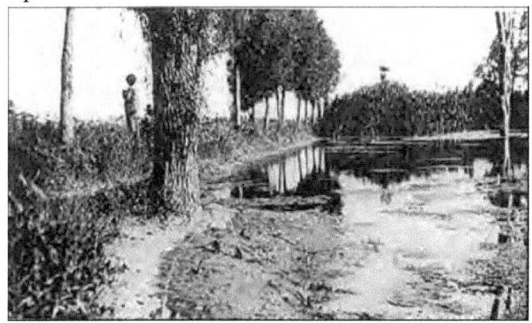

Photo N° 2. Floating masses of algae on one side of the lake, behind the dam; important *Anopheles pseudopunctipennis* breeding site. Cañitas Viejo, Ledesma; Jujuy, (9).

They also claimed that the favorable larval development depended largely on the existence of algae, at least for the occurrence of a large production of these mosquitoes.

From the epidemiological point of view, they considered two malaria areas of unequal importance in Argentina. The most important one covered the northwestern provinces, including Jujuy, Salta and Tucuman, and small towns in the east of the provinces of Catamarca and La Rioja, north of San Luis, northwestern Córdoba and along Dulce River in Santiago del Estero, up to the city of Santiago, where this type of malaria also occurred. These regions coincided with the distribution of *An. pseudopunctipennis* (except San Luis, where no specimens had been collected); this species had been confirmed to be the most important vector in this country; hence, we can assume that the prevalence of malaria in northern Argentina depended mainly on the presence of this species. The other area, of less importance, was along Bermejo, Paraná and Paraguay rivers, comprising riparian areas of these rivers in the provinces of Corrientes, Santa Fe, Chaco, Formosa and Misiones. Those authors did not know about the presence of *pseudopunctipennis* in the area and assumed there would be other species of the genus *Anopheles* belonging to the *Nysshorynchus* group (*albitarsis, argyritarsis* and *tarsimaculatus*) that may be involved in transmission; moreover, it was possible that along the Bermejo River, in the Chaco, part of malaria would be transmitted by *An. pseudopunctipennis*.

In the following years, there was little impact of Paterson's findings and there were other research contributions, such as that of Carlos Alvarado, (13) and of Juana Petrocchi, who drew similar conclusions by studying northwestern mosquitoes, (9). In previous years, Alois Bachman, Chief of malaria of Famaillá, Tucumán, had published his findings about mosquitoes and determined the usual *An. pseudopunctipennis* microenvironment in the local environment (14). Despite these conclusions, the DNH indicated advances in the 1928 control program in a progress report about malaria control, claiming the benefits of wetland drainage at a large scale in the city and surrounding areas: through engineering works they had created a comprehensive network of drainage canals and hydraulic regularization of Famaillá.

Such works were examples of *piccola bonifica*. The malaria service sanitation work, however, barely treated the Famaillá river banks, where Bachman found *An pseudopunctipennis* breeding sites in infiltration areas. It was notable that, despite the evidence, it was difficult to go against the prevailing trend in the endemic control strategy.

In 1937, a phase of qualitative advances began with the identification of the population and the surface area corresponding to the malaria endemic zone of northwestern Argentina. Accordingly, a special protagonist, Dr. Carlos Alberto Alvarado, was the driver of the effective transformation of control activities in Argentina. He understood that Europe's control measures, transferred without proper adaptation to the prevailing vector bionomics, were probably the reason for the failure of the applied health efforts.

In 1937, already appointed chief of the General Directorate of Malaria, created by Act of Congress, in Tucumán Dr. Alvarado was in charge of malaria control for the entire country. His working methods included the following fundamental aspects:

"Foci patrol" plan, intended to eliminate anopheline breeding sites at a distance of four kilometers from the protected area. This strategy was based on local findings in the province of Jujuy. He and his colleagues found numerous *An. pseudopunctipennis* larvae in irrigation infiltration areas and a network of canals crossing Rio Grande River, as well as nearby canals and springs. These sites tended to be populated exclusively by one species or another (either *An. pseudopunctipennis* or *An. argyritarsis*), but could be only meters away from one another along the same river or canal. Alvarado indicates that some *An. pseudopunctipennis* larvae were found in canals or streams, with straight steep banks, relatively free of vegetation, except for a surface layer of *Spyrogira* algae, whereas a*rgyritarsis*, and not p*seudopunctipennis*, were found in streams with irregular banks and abundant aquatic vegetation. These associations between the two species of mosquitoes and their respective microenvironments became so obvious that, when taking the larva samples to the laboratory, the field workers were able to identify the species, almost always correctly, depending on collection site (15). He found a temporary stream formed in spring that had been previously cleaned; he had it straightened and deepened in sanitation works populated by numerous *An. pseudopunctipennis* larvae. He named the stream modified as re-naturalized. Workers straightened the windings of the beds of irrigation channels and / or streams with picks and shovels, aquatic vegetation was transplanted and the stream bed was expanded, thus exposing it to the shade of trees and shrubs along the banks. This area was left untreated, and was soon populated by *argyritarsis* larvae, whereas *pseudopunctipennis* left the site. It was clear that these algae determined the *An. pseudopunctipennis* growing area. Based on this, plus the collection of field observations and evidence from the literature, Alvarado determined that it was the algae, and not the water temperature or water chemistry, the factor presenting the key explanatory variable. Those sites where *spirogyra* algae dominated were also occupied by *pseudopunctipennis* larvae. If these algae were absent, they would be replaced by large aquatic plants, and so would be *pseudopunctipennis* larvae.

Alvarado exposed the field observations and the influence of what he called re-naturalization of watercourses, which was exactly the opposite of what was being done at the time: allow the influence of suitable vegetation in channels that would compete with *spirogyra*, and that under most circumstances, during the growing season a biological equilibrium would be established, which meant the prevalence of other plants and heavy algae presence, (15). As a result, *pseudopunctipennis* larvae production would decrease, whereas other species of Anopheles would occupy places with more mature vegetation. "After testing several hypotheses, Alvarado postulated that for the development of their larvae, *An. pseudopunctipennis* needs absence of vertical aquatic vegetation, well ventilated, sunlit and constantly renewed waters and the presence of *spirogirae* algae which provides food and shelter. These phenomena were facilitated by the hydraulic *bonifica* or the *piccola bonifica*. The proposed solution was to 're-naturalize' waterways by planting watercress, *Nasturtium officinale,* and "lampazo", *Cenesio cremeiphlorum Matti,* in the bed, and shrubs and / or trees for shade on the margins, such as privets, *Ligustrum japonicum,* golden willow, *Salix vitallina*; and poplars of different varieties like willow beach, *Salix humboldtiana*, and white willow, *Salix alba*. The result was the disappearance of *An pseudopunctipennis* larvae", (6,7,16).

Imbuido con el nuevo conocimiento del microambiente de los mosquitos, esta estrategia se ocupaba de los siguientes elementos:

Convinced that larva removal depended on the control of alga growth and based on the value of a year of experiments, Alvarado reoriented the campaign to what he called "foci police ", or "foci patrol", (15,16). With the contribution of the recently gained knowledge of mosquito microenvironment, this strategy addressed the following items:

1. The finding, treatment and / or elimination of the sources of *An. Pseudopunctipennis* growth, especially through the removal of algae. Workers physically removed mats of algae from streams / ditches with picks, shovels, hoes and brooms; and where it was less feasible to remove the seaweed, they treated growing areas with oil or Paris Green (copper aceto-arsenite). This strategy led to immediate quantifieble results. The blood rate of people in La Viña in the province of Jujuy, only by applying this methodology and without the administration of quinine, fell from 30% in April 1929 to 7.3% in October 1934. In November 1933, 73 *An. pseudopunctipennis* were collected from 14 homes; a year later only 2 adults were collected from 19 households, (ibid).

With the "foci patrol" strategy, Alvarado's program represented an important break with the conventional sanitation used until then. This experience was the support for future actions of the malaria control program in Argentina, until the advent of the campaign with DDT.

2. The winter prophylaxis, which was used with the arrival of cold weather, which consisted of sterilizing an increasingly wide radius and preventing vector breeding in the area.

3. Quinine administration to populations of unprotected areas, even if they were far away.

Control of results, measured by various methods (hematological index, spleen index, anopheles index) showed the program effectiveness. In a few years, the Malaria Directorate studied the extension and identified the endemic regional characteristics, created the most effective and low-cost methods to combat the disease, studied new anti-malarial drugs, built anti-larval water siphons, cultivated larvae-eating fish, established the role of rice fields in the spread of anopheles, and fundamentally, worked on health education among the local people exposed to the risk of infection, (5,8,16).

Littoral epidemic malaria was also studied; the capital cities as well as some localities of the provinces of Tucumán, Jujuy, Salta and Catamarca were protected. The approach in rural areas, where it was not possible to implement these procedures due to the lack of resources, was the distribution of specific medication.

3. SECOND PHASE
1940 – 1949

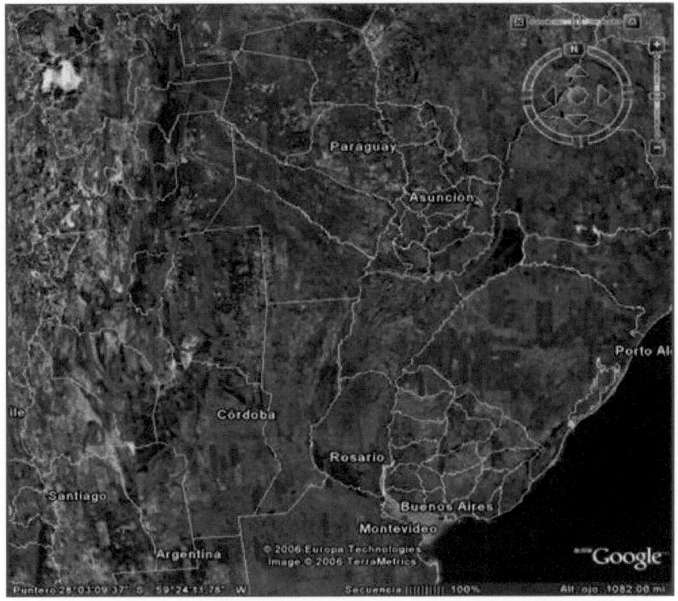

Figure N° 5. 1940. Malaria endemic area in Argentina, (PNP)

A limited analysis of the epidemiological situation in Argentina in those years clearly showed two scenarios already outlined by different researchers: one in the northwest and another in the northeast of the country, (17).

The scenario in the northwest (NOA) covered the Andean and pre-Andean foothills, with an estimated area of 120,000 km², and included the provinces of Salta, Jujuy, Tucuman, Catamarca, La Rioja and foci in Santiago del Estero, northeast of Cordoba, San Juan, and a population of 850,000 inhabitants. The prevailing vector in the area was *Anopheles pseudopunctipennis*, showing a severe endemic expression.

In northeastern Argentina (NEA) there was an epidemic malaria strip with small endemic foci, caused by epidemic extensions from neighboring countries that affected the provinces of Misiones, Corrientes, Chaco, Formosa and Santa Fe, also covering an area of approximately 120,000 km². The vector identified in the area was *Anopheles darlingi.*

In 1946, the government created the National Ministry of Public Health and Social Welfare (formerly Secretariat), headed by Dr. Ramon Carrillo. The Analytical Public Health Plan is developed, implementing administrative decentralization (creating general directorates of Health). Alvarado was appointed General Director of Malaria and Tropical Diseases of the Public Health Ministry in September 1947. In that year, Alvarado submitted a plan of action at the request of the recently appointed minister, which consisted in spraying with DDT (dichlorodiphenyltrichloroethane) houses in more than 120,000 km² in endemic areas and a similar amount at those sites where the disease appeared temporarily. Available staff is increased and a project of "DDT fumigation" that was part of the First Five-Year Plan of Government is programmed, which consisted of the arrival of a truck fleet to Tucuman intended to "eradicate malaria", (18,19). The planned strategy was based on the particular anthropophilic and endophagous habits of the vector, *An pseudopunctipennis*, with the chances of success of the campaign relying on this knowledge. And the plan success could be achieved according to the possibilities of execution, as well as the methodology to be used, (16).

The latter instance had to be decided by the technicians who faced a challenge, since vector elimination campaigns implied at least eight years (one year for the preparatory phase, four years for the attack phase and three years for consolidation). The preparatory phase consisted of the accurate geographical recognition of the area, operational planning and service organization, and human resources. As the new plan was conceived, it implied a true operational revolution that required an unknown speed of actions and a dynamics that would effectively facilitate vector removal from the treatment areas. Sixteen of the twenty sanitation services installed were removed in the first year of work, and the remaining four in the second, on the grounds that new achievements would justify that action. Suspended works included anti-larval measures taken in peri-urban areas, (18).

Works with DDT were fulfilled with 70 mobile brigades operating in an area of approximately 150.00 km². Each brigade had an area to cover, and they were composed of two or three sprayers, depending on whether they would work in urban or rural areas. Each one was able to spray on average 3,500 homes per year, with variable performance in rural or urban areas, and each one had a chief responsible for the activity, (ibid). In the first campaign sprayings were performed every three months, in the second every four months and in the third every five months. The activity schedule depended on the epidemiological variability of malaria in endemic areas; transmission period in the NOA was considered shorter according to the monitoring of detection of diseased persons and adult anopheline captures, using data from the ten years preceding the campaign with DDT. The climate was also considered, since in summer rains made many rural roads impassable; staff and equipment available: and the estimated residual properties, which at that time were five months for DDT and three months for benzene hexachloride. Work started in sparsely populated areas, and involved house spraying in bedrooms, living rooms, kitchens, bathrooms, etc.; thus, the effectiveness was considered to be ensured in a treatment that was mostly influenced by the time it took to get to the houses, (ibid).

Once the rural areas were covered, urban areas were treated, but in a centripetal way, from outside inwards, in a "crown" mode, spraying a belt of between 5 and 8 blocks around the city center, in an attempt to include the range of the vector. In 1947, the first year of the campaign, 40% of the malaria endemic area was intended to be covered. In the second year, 80% of the area was planned, with estimates being made based on the population (and not on the land area) (16).

The operation logistics appeared as a major obstacle considering that vehicles had to travel by all kinds of roads and paths, many of them impassable, and staff had to spend the night in isolated spots, where the necessary fuel and supplies should be available, (ibid). Urban areas were treated in a centripetal mode, by applying DDT on a delimited belt several blocks wide in the peripheral area of each locality. Thus, a barrier of several hundred meters of urban area covered with sprayed houses was established. During the first year several difficulties were faced, such as the lack of the necessary vehicles and sufficient fuel tanks as well as the low number of professional engineers who technically handled spraying of houses; all these factors were critical for the implementation of the activities in the field, (18).

Development: The new plan was aimed to cover 40% of the endemic area (expressed in malarial population and not in surface area) in 1947. In 1948, the plan was expanded to 80%, which intended to eliminate four-fifths of malaria in two years. (16)

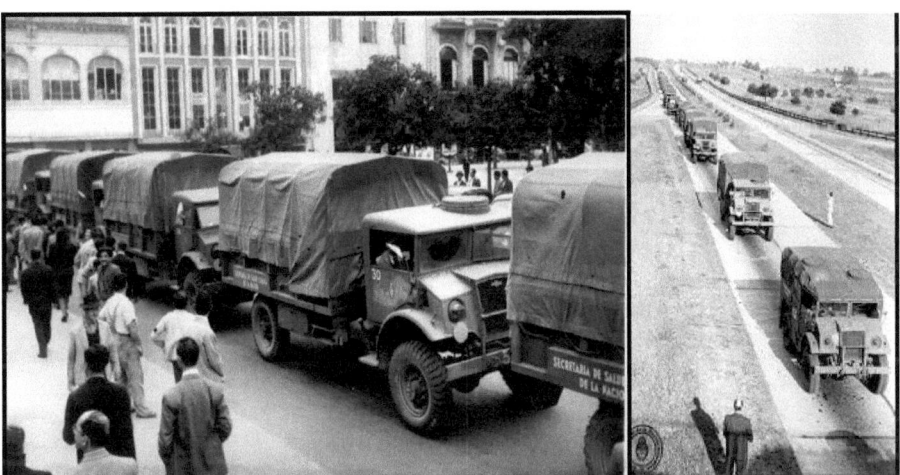

Photos Nº 3 and 4. Group of motor vehicles of the Ministry of Health during the DDT fumigation campaign.

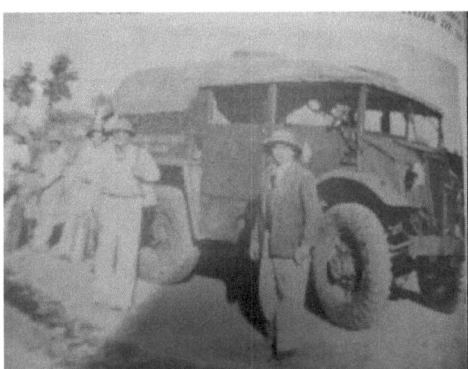

Photo Nº. 5. Fumigation team, 1948

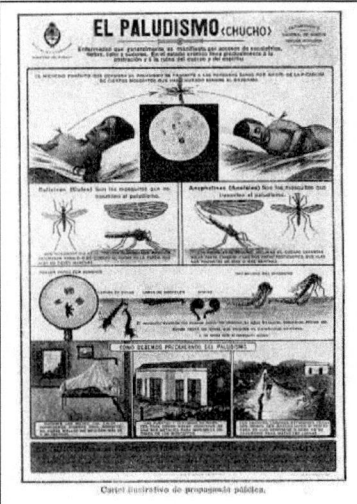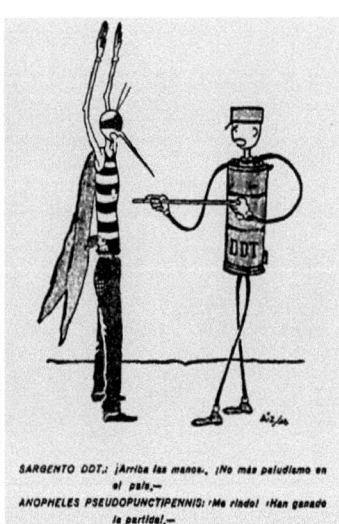

Figures N° 5 and 6. Dissemination material about malaria for public sites, schools, offices.

Annual vector spread in the regions was not uniform in the endemic area; it showed a progressive downward north to south trend. Then spraying was planned to be conducted in two weeks before the appearance of the first adults in the region. The schedule was the following. Two cycles were planned in the northern part of the northwest endemic areas and in Misiones, because the transmission period was six to eight months. In the southern part of the northwest endemic area, where the transmission period was less than six months, one cycle would be conducted.

Thus, Argentina was the first country in the Americas to use DDT spraying as a routine procedure, thereby abandoning the "foci patrol" plan. The appearance of DDT and other residual insecticides introduced new elements to the strategic concept of malaria control and modified techniques existing until then in its fundamental aspects, known as the theater of operations, strategic objective, economic base and cost estimates, (18, 19).

From January 1949 to the end of July of that year, 802 cases were recorded all throughout the endemic area. Argentina significantly reduced the endemic malaria to several hundred cases, and the principles guiding malaria control and procedures that were implemented served as a model for other countries. Argentine legislation on malaria control was considered to be the most complete and effective of the rules existing on that subject.

As it had been originally planned, the health care plan would be transformed into surveillance service. The conversion is based on the need to train personnel in epidemiological surveillance activities. The main activity of the personnel included: 1) detection and capture of anopheles in fumigated surfaces and 2) investigation of all malaria cases that may occur in the area.

This surveillance service was composed of staff of various levels and from different work sites: doctors from other government agencies, hospitals, schools, school teachers, factory managers, camps foremen and a volunteer network. The purpose was also to communicate cases of malaria of which they were aware. In all opportunities the corresponding documentary piece should be attached, which consisted of the plate or slide with blood smear; for this, the microscopist was an essential member of the staff. The alert service was organized as a consolidation phase of the anti-malaria strategy.

The basic components of the strategy proposed since then consisted of implementing a program for epidemiological surveillance, with three elements:
1. Research: passive and active detection, epidemiological research after confirmation of the case, classification of cases and monitoring of positive cases.
2. Healing: presumptive, radical and mass treatment.
3. Environmental control: spraying of houses.

This strategy contributed to a radical decrease in the number of cases in the following years.

YEARS	NORTH COUNTRY TOTAL	CENTRAL AND COASTAL COUNTRY	GENERAL TOTAL COUNTRY	HOUSE SPRAYING	DDT CONSUMED (Kilogram)	PROTECTED POPULATION
1947	40,772	2,240	43,012	560	889	3,341
1948	15,025	1,077	16,102			
1949	3,080	195	3,275			
1950	639	1,323	1,962	35,779	36,994	246,993
1951	312	1,021	1,333			
1952	563	133	696			
1953	428	71	499			
1954	401	23	424	174,067		104,000
1955	331	3	334		146,299	

Source: Bulletin of the Pan American Sanitary Bureau, vol. XL, n° 3 March 1956, 258 and 259.

Table N° 2. Malaria cases recorded from July 1947 to July 1955

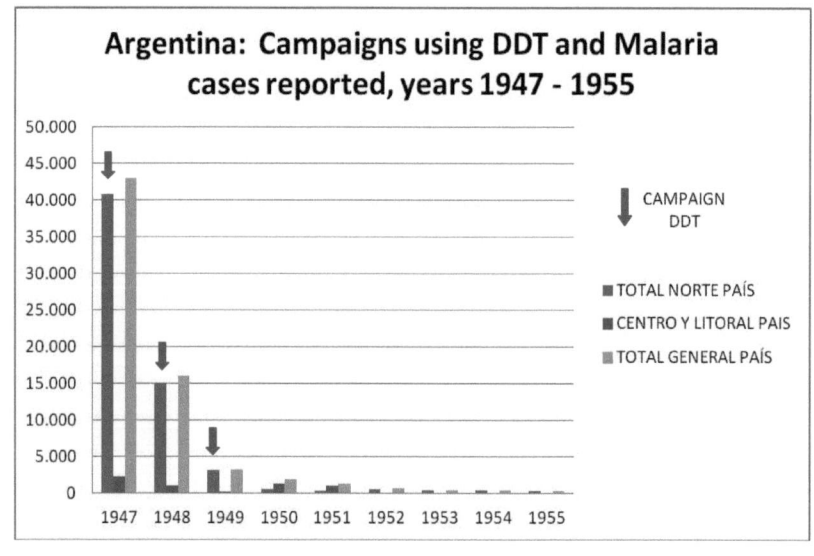

Figure N°. 8. Evolution of case records during the years of campaign, 1947-1949 and six years post-intervention, 1950-1955. Source: Bol.de la Oficina Sanitaria Panamericana, vol. XL, n° 3, March 1956, pp. 258 y 259.

In late 1949, Dr. Alvarado stated: "We have finished with endemic malaria, but the struggle continues by systematically spraying all the houses in the endemic area every four months. Works are directed by our anti-malarial Engineering Department; all classic engineering work has been interrupted to deal exclusively with DDT-spraying", (16).

Although no post-intervention infestation rates were obtained, the evidence was that *An. pseudopunctipennis* larvae were detected only through a thorough search of the vector and that it was not possible to identify adult individuals (ibid).

Since this achievement, and already in 1949, in just over a year, all field activities were carried out by different types of collaborators, including doctors, teachers, rural workers, and a network of officious collaborators who participated in the epidemiological malaria Surveillance tasks. The work consisted of DDT spraying of the area, monitoring of existing breeding sites, entomological evaluation of housing and detection of patients suspected of malaria, whereas in the non-sprayed area, the emergence of cases was monitored and healthcare was provided.

4. THIRD PHASE
1950 – 2008

The strategy proposed since the previous decade basically consisted of the establishment of a program to conduct epidemiological surveillance, with three components:

1. Research: passive and active detection, epidemiological research after confirmation of the case, classification of cases and monitoring of positive cases.
2. Healing: presumptive, radical and mass treatment.
3. Environmental control: house spraying.

Surveillance activities were basically conducted in the updated risk zone. Thus, the areas to be covered were selected according to the occurrence of cases in the last two years, (Technical Report PNP, 2008).

The program includes visits to the houses, following a fixed, predefined route, where the following activities were routinely performed:

a. Family censuses,
b. Detection of febrile cases,
c. Fingerstick blood collection,
d. Entomological evaluation of the site.

If a suspected patient was detected, blood samples were taken not only from the patient but also from cohabitants and neighbors living near the patient's house. The blood sample was transported to the operational base, where there was the necessary equipment for microscopic diagnosis; there, samples were stained and read. If the case was positive, epidemiological assessment of the case was completed and specific standardized medication was administered. Then the patient's house and neighboring houses were sprayed with residual pyrethroid insecticides.

This approach strategy still remains in full force, with some non-significant operational variations.

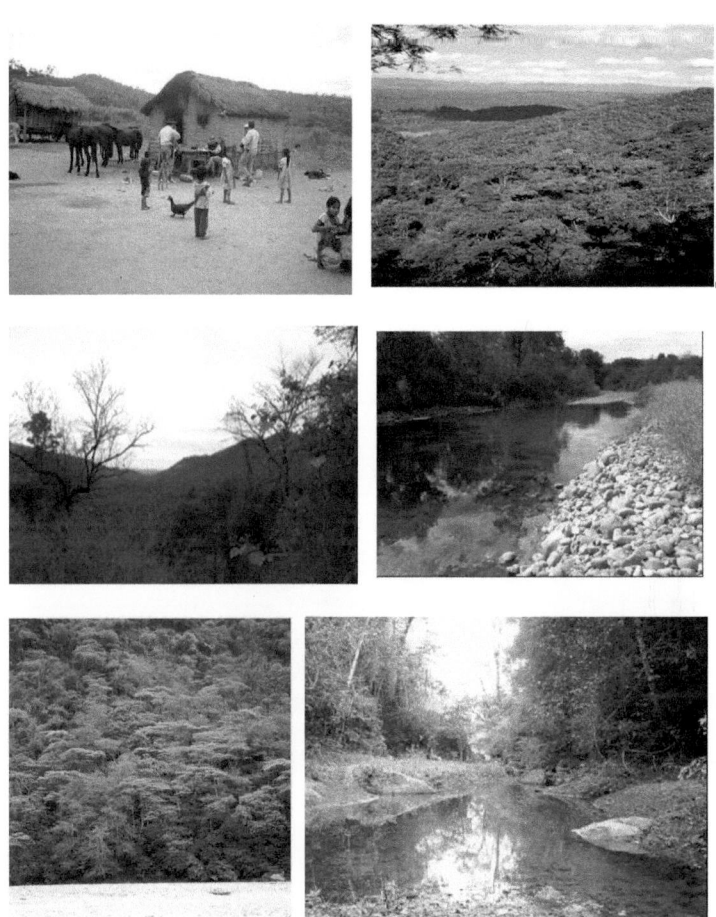

Photos N°.6, 7, 8, 9, 10, 11. Diverse habitats of endemic across northwestern Argentina

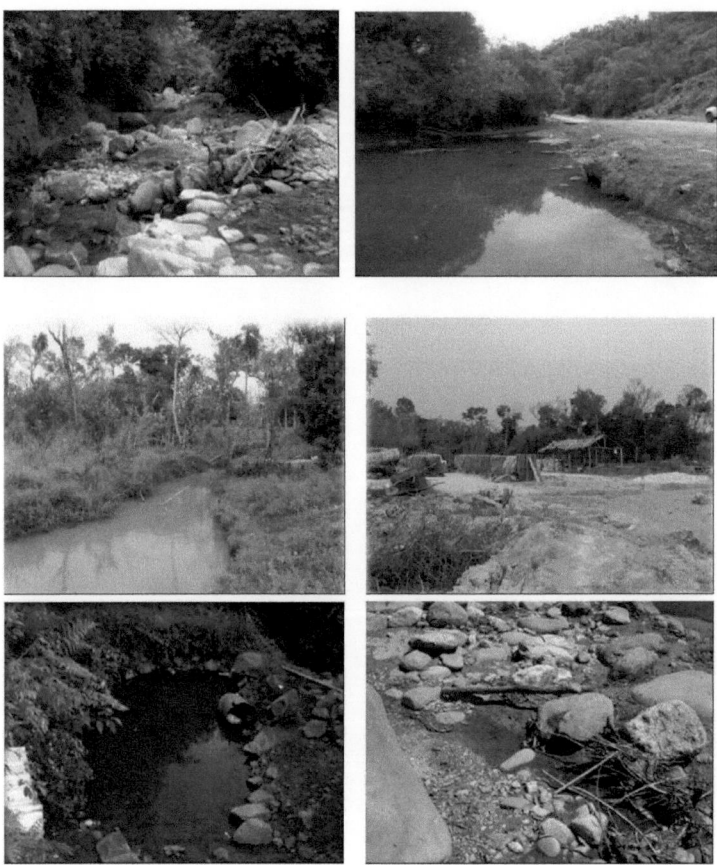

Photos N°. 12,13,14,15,16,17. Other habitats of the endemic area.

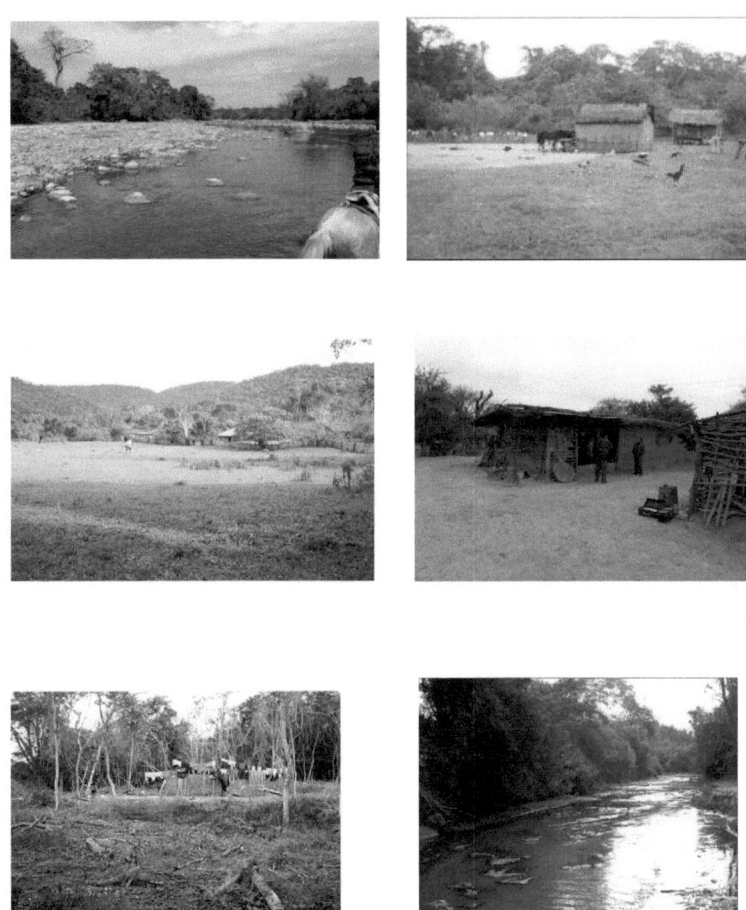

Photos N°. 18, 19, 20, 21, 22, 23. North western endemic area.

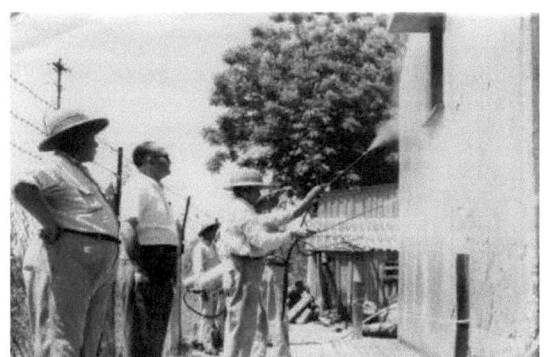

Photo N°24. P.A.H.O. officials observing team members applying residual insecticide in a practical demonstration, year 1960.

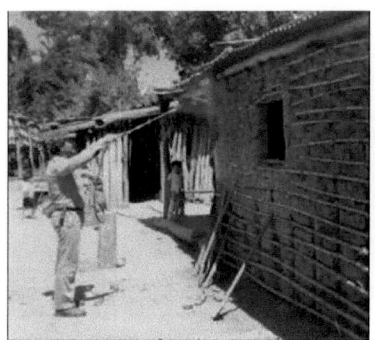 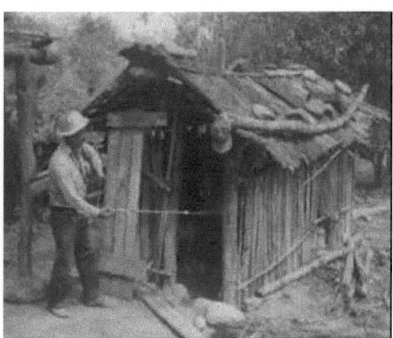

Photos N°. 25 and 26: Members of the crew spraying in the field, year 1970

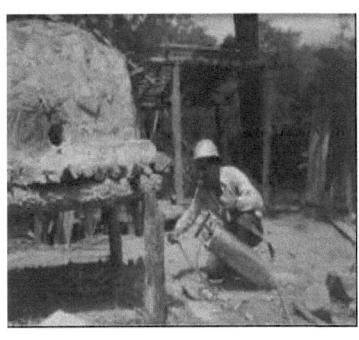 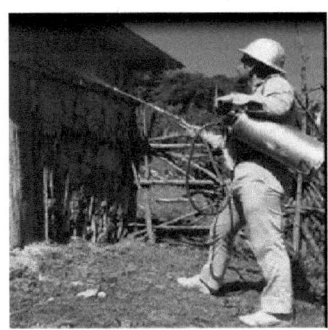

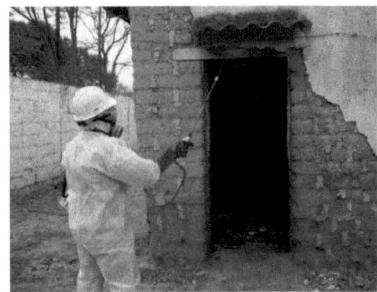 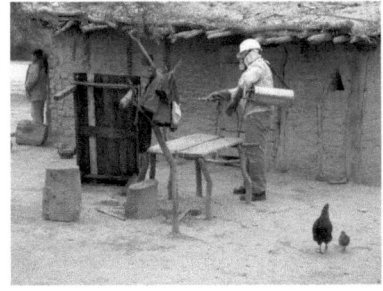

Photos N° 27, 28, 29, 30: Technical spraying at different times, 1970, and 2010.

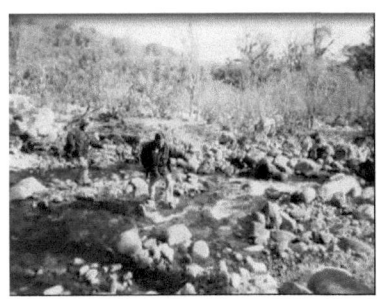 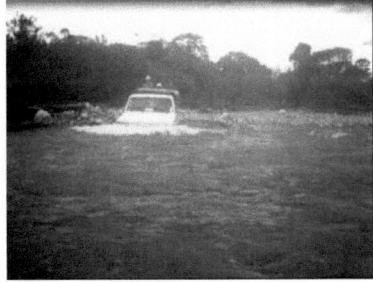

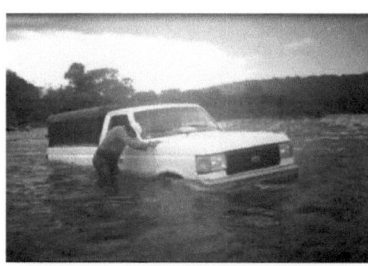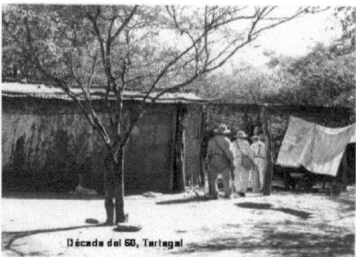

Photos N° 31, 32 33, 34. Staff movement and rivers crossing in the work area vicinity, Oran department. The last photo is from the year 60 in Tartagal, malaria endemic area, Salta.

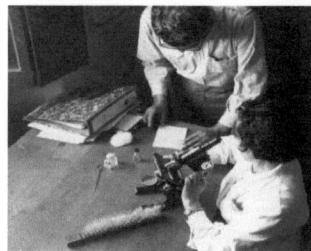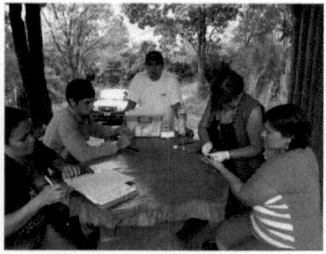

Photos N° 35 and 36. Personnel performing evaluation tasks and blood sampling in the area of Palma Sola, Jujuy(1965) and Puerto Iguazú, Misiones, 2014.

Entomological studies

In the late 50s, Dr Juan Bejarano described the situation of that time based on updated findings of prevalent anopheles in NOA and NEA, (21). He depicted *An. pseudopunctipennis* breeding sites as: primary natural breeding sites (rivers and streams), sectors exposed to sunlight, clear water, slow water flow containing filamentous green algae; secondary or expansion breeding sites: in lakes, springs and other flooded areas exposed to the sun with or without algae: tertiary, or exception breeding sites, swamps, bogs, etc. Artificial breeding sites: dams, canals, drains, rice fields, pools, deposits, etc. The species flight radius was established at about 6 kilometers; primary breeding sites were found up to an altitude of 2200 meters, as in Punta Balastro, Catamarca. Malarial infection was studied and oocyst rate of 2.1% and a sporozoite rate of 0.86% were detected, (2305 samples); the southernmost distribution was San Francisco in the province of San Luis (32° 40' S). He emphasized that *An pseudopunctipennis* occurred in and near mountain areas and that it had high density, domesticity and anthropophily, and low infectivity, resulting a quantitative transmitter. At that time, some points were still uncertain, such as species survival during the cold months of severe winter weather. Regarding the systematics, Dr Bejarano concluded that it was a complex of several subspecies or varieties.

He concluded that it was possible to accept that the biological knowledge about *Anopheles (A.) pseudopunctipennis (s.l.)* allowed Alvarado and colleagues to plan the fight against the winged forms using intradomiciliary DDT spraying. Thus, malaria ceased to be the serious socioeconomic health problem that had been for the provinces of northwestern Argentina until then.

Regarding vectors from northeastern Argentina, since the earliest descriptions, two anopheles were particularly important in malaria epidemiology in the area: *An albitarsis* and *An darling;* the latter specimen seems more domiciliary and anthropophilic than para-Andean specimens. They were detected inside rooms occupied by people in the localities of Curuzu Cuatia, Yapeyú, Pueblo Galarza, Estancia San Solano and Colonia Pellegrini, in Corrientes province. Del Ponte indicated that *An albitarsis* did not breed in pond waters in the rice fields and malarial plasmodium infection had not been determined until then. The species has been attributed to malaria transmission in some outbreaks in the provinces of Chaco, Santa Fe and Corrientes, between 1939 and 1940, (22).

An darlingi was found in Puerto Bemberg, Eldorado and San Pedro, (Misiones). In 1946 during an intense epidemic affecting Puerto Iguazu and extented to Posadas, capital city of the province, breeding sites were detected in streams in Puerto Iguazu and Eldorado and even in rafts in Puerto Bemberg. Lifshitz, Umana and Vergara, (23), demonstrated that *An darlingi* specimens captured in Puerto Iguazu, Iguazu Cue, Puerto Bemberg and Puerto Eldorado were infected with malaria. Specimens were detected in 79 homes; 90 of the specimens were *darlingi*, 4 *noroestensis* and 1 *holmsbergi*.

Evolution of control

With the above mentioned strategy, a gradual and steady decline occurred in the provinces considered endemic until the end of the 60s (1969), when most provinces showed no new cases, except for Salta and Jujuy, which continued with a persistent endemic level, especially in Salta, over the years and sporadic outbreaks occurrences in Misiones province, (17, 24).

Since that time, the occurrence of cases was mainly characterized by migration flows in the area of Argentine-Bolivian border. This complex environment involves southern Tarija department in Bolivia, and northern Salta, in Oran and San Martin departments. This area has ecological conditions (tropical climate with wet season and extreme temperature and high humidity with seasonal variations) as well as social and entomological conditions (presence of various anopheles in the area, as well as *Aedes aegypti* and *Triatoma infestans*, Dengue and Chagas vectors).

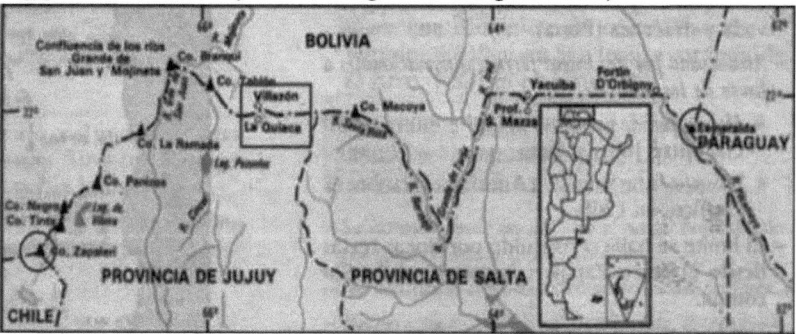

Figure N° 9. Argentine-Bolivian border area. It extends from the Cerro Zapaleri on the western end to Hito Esmeraldas on the eastern end, Argentine-Bolivian-Paraguayan tripoint.

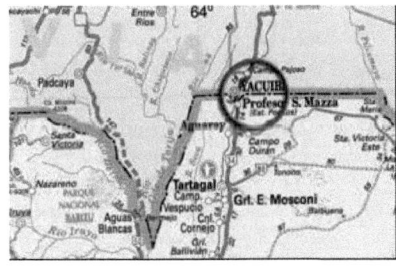 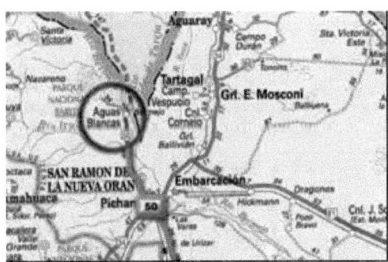

Fig. N°. 10 and 11. Argentine border sites of Malaria epidemiological importance. Top left: border with Bolivia, (Bermejo) on Oran and Aguas Blancas. Top right: border with Bolivia (Yacuiba) in Salvador Mazza.

Population movements on both border sides are intense, with prevailing north-south direction, usually for work purposes. They generally involve people moving with their family group to work in the harvest of cotton, sugarcane and fruit and vegetable crops in the northern provinces of Argentina, (17, 24). People enter the country both through officially authorized border crossings and numerous informal passages along the 742-km long frontier, (National Geographic Institute). The border is demarcated on the west end by Cerro Zapaleri, tripartite point of Argentina, Bolivia and Chile.

Argentina borders with Paraguay along 500 km on the east and is characterized by areas with occurrence of malarial transmission in the last decades. To the west, the frontier is characterized by topographic relief of more than 3000 in height, in Bermejo and Toldo regions; then, to the southeast, the frontier extends up to Fortin Campero at the confluence of Bermejo and Grande de Tarija rivers, area known as La Juntas de San Antonio. Then the frontier continues up along the Grande de Tarija and Itáu rivers, up to the locality of Yacuiba. From this locality, the frontier follows the parallel 22°S to the east up to Fortin D'Orbigny on Pilcomayo river, and along this river up to Hito Esmeralda, the tripartite point between Argentina, Paraguay and Bolivia. (25).

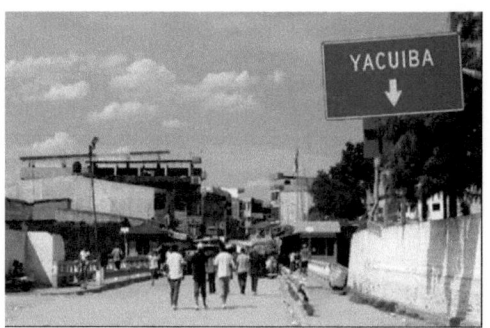

Photo N° 35: People travelling from Argentina to Bolivia on the International Bridge linking Salvador Mazza with Pocitos, Yacuiba, Bolivia.

Along the border, there are "mirror" populations, such as Bermejo (B) and Aguas Blancas (A); Yacuiba (B) and Salvador Mazza (A), where large migration flows establish in the malaria endemic area (La Quiaca - Villazón are not included because they do not belong to the endemic area). There are also informal crossing points along this border where mostly rural workers enter and settle illegally or without having the required documents. Their stay in the country becomes difficult; in addition, there is the risk of patients that migrate during the disease incubation period and then, when the first symptoms appear, resort to traditional healers or pharmacies seeking medication for their fever process. Only when any complications appear or when the symptoms do not disappear with medication, do these people seek services or go to health centers for the necessary attention, (24). An additional complication in the border area is related to the movement of people linked to the activity of smuggling of goods such as clothing and household items, and illegal goods such as cocaine; therefore, violent incidents related to this situation and their consequent derivations have occurred in the area in recent years.

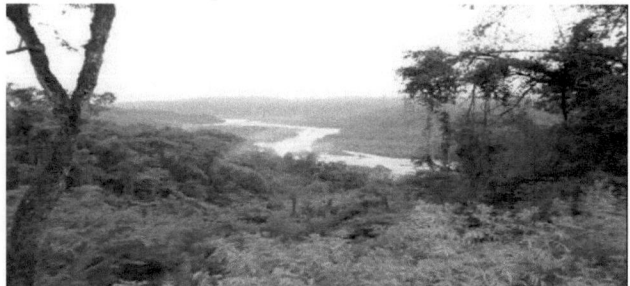

Photo N° 36,. Endemic area in the Yungas, Oran department.

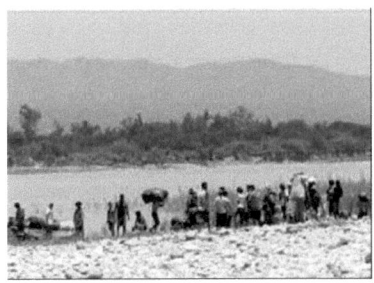 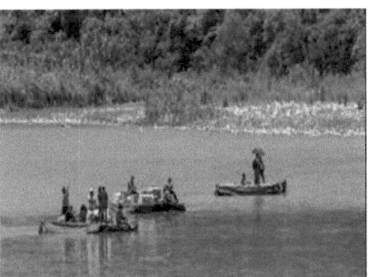

Photos N° 37, 38, 39 . People carrying different goods on Bermejo river, Argentine - Bolivian border.

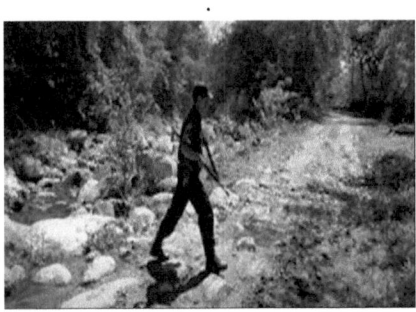

Photo N° 40: . Gendarme crossing a gravel road at the border, locality of S. Mazza, Argentine border.

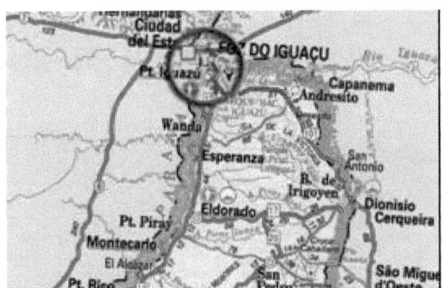

Figure N° 12. Triple frontier in the northeast, Paraguay (Ciudad del Este), Foz do Iguazú (Brazil) and Puerto Iguazú (Misiones, Argentina).

Today, in Argentina the area corresponding to Puerto Iguazú department is a residual malarial area. This department is located in the northwest corner of the province of Misiones, Argentina. It borders the departments of Eldorado, General Manuel Belgrano and the countries of Brazil and Paraguay, forming the Triple Border. The department has a 2,736 km² area, representing 9.21% of the total province. Its population is 82,227 (according to the 2010 INDEC census). It also has a strong recent trend of immigration from the Paraguayan and Brazilian borders. An unknown number of residents that come from Paraguay and Brazil have not been recorded in the census. As a frontier area, intense migratory movements related to tourism, trade and local border traffic occur. Technical reports of the corresponding offices of the respective Ministries of Health (Ministry of Health of the State of Parana, Brazil and SENEPA, Paraguay, National Malaria Elimination Plan Paraguay, 2011 – 2015, March 2011 National Malaria Control Program SENEPA), indicate a negative record of new indigenous cases in the last couple of years on both borders.

For more than seven years, no indigenous cases have been recorded in the department of Puerto Iguazú, (Technical report PNP, 2014).

Contemporary entomological studies
Northwestern Argentina

In the early 2000s, after the last works that referred to the presence of anopheles mosquitoes in the NOA and NEA in the 70s, there was a long period without any new contributions of the knowledge of Anopheles species present in localities with records of malaria transmission, as well as of the characteristics of potential/s vector/s of malaria in northwestern Argentina. Various entomological studies significantly contributed to the understanding of the dynamics of the main malaria vector, *An pseudopunctipennis*, in the endemic area of the country.

Thus, from December 2001 to December 2005, various investigations aimed at performing bio-ecological studies of anopheline mosquitoes in two areas of the Yungas: Orán department, Salta province (north area of the Yungas), and Monteros department, Tucumán province (south area of the Yungas). The selected localities were: Aguas Blancas, El Oculto and San Ramón de la Nueva Orán (northern area) and Capitán Cáceres, La Florida and Sargento Moya (southern area).

When these studies on anopheline mosquitoes began, *An. pseudopunctipennis* seasonal distribution and the influence of climatic variables in a known malarial area in northern

Salta had been preliminarily analyzed for one year. Three environments were differentiated at the selected location: forest, forest edge and peridomicile. The results showed that *An. pseudopunctipennis* was the most abundant species, as well as the presence of other species, such as *An. strodei* and *An. argyritarsis*. At the same time, *An. pseudopunctipennis* was captured throughout the year but its greatest abundance was between September and December (spring). Finally, the average maximum humidity was the variable of greatest influence on the seasonal abundance of species, (26).

In a second work, the abundance of *Anopheles* species collected from different environments (forest, forest edge and peridomicile), was analyzed to explore how environmental differences affect the spatial distribution of these mosquitoes. Again, *An. pseudopunctipennis* was found to be the most abundant species, with *An. argyritarsis*, *An. rangeli* and *An. strodei* being also collected. In addition, while all species were collected from the three environments, the highest abundance of anopheles was found in the forest edge, (27).

Subsequent studies focused on exploring the relationships between the distribution and abundance of anopheline mosquitoes and climatic conditions and environmental changes. Data on the Normalized Difference Vegetation Index (NDVI) and Surface Temperature (LST) were obtained from Moderate Resolution Imaging Spectroradiometer (MODIS) as well as climatic factors (temperature, humidity, wind speed and accumulated precipitation) from gauging stations. Mosquitoes were captured from three locations, Aguas Blancas, El Oculto and San Ramón de la Nueva Orán, in an area of malaria transmission north of the Yungas. Most anopheline mosquitoes were collected from El Oculto town and to a lesser extent from Aguas Blancas and San Ramón de la Nueva Orán. The most abundant species were *Anopheles pseudopunctipennis* in El Oculto, *Anopheles argyritarsis* in Aguas Blancas and *Anopheles strodei* in San Ramón de la Nueva Orán. The specimens were collected during the four years of capture, with the highest peaks of abundance being in spring. Surface temperature and average temperature were the variables that determined the distribution patterns and the greatest abundance of *An. pseudopunctipennis* and *An. argyritarsis* within the malarial area, (28).

The separate study of the temporal and spatial fluctuation of the main vector involved in malaria transmission, *An. pseudopunctipennis* and the potential vector *An. argyritarsis* in the two areas of Yungas from northwestern Argentina showed that former species was more abundant in the northern area of the Yungas, whereas *An. argyritarsis* was more abundant in the southern area. In turn, *An. pseudopunctipennis* showed high abundance in spring, which has important epidemiological implications in the northern area (since the first cases of malaria appear in this season) and although the role of *An. argyritarsis* in Malaria transmission is still questioned, it is important to note that its high abundance in both study areas was in spring. Finally, climatic factors determining the greatest abundance of these two species were mean maximum and minimum temperatures, (29).

In a study of malaria transmission in two localities where disease transmission was both autochthonous and imported, on the border with Bolivia, *An. pseudopunctipennis* was found to be the dominant species in El Oculto (where only autochthonous transmission was reported) but not in Aguas Blancas (where both modes of transmission were). *Anopheles pseudopunctipennis* showed a seasonal continuous distribution over time, but in Aguas Blancas, a marked seasonality with peaks in late spring and early summer was observed. Mean maximum temperature and mean maximum humidity were associated with the fluctuation of *An. pseudopunctipennis* for both localities. Regarding the disease, mean maximum temperature was associated with an increase in malaria cases in El Oculto whereas in Aguas Blancas, mean temperature was the most significant variable.

It should be noted that in Aguas Blancas, the peak of vector abundance in late spring and early summer was related to the appearance of malaria cases three months later, i.e., in summer and autumn, (30).

A longitudinal study focused on species composition and temporal and spatial abundance of *Anopheles* larvae in a malaria transmission risk area in northwestern Argentina analyzed the influence of environmental factors on population dynamics. Sampling included different types of aquatic habitats such as pools, irrigation canals, ponds and mountain streams, located both in suburban areas of the locality of San Ramón de la Nueva Orán and in mountain rivers in El Oculto and ravines near Aguas Blancas, north of the province of Salta. First, it was observed that the immature forms of this genus reproduce mainly in water bodies that have certain bio-ecological characteristics, such as some degree of oxygenation, slow flowing waters, and especially the presence of green algae. The most abundant captured species was *An. Pseudopunctipennis*, followed by *An. argyritarsis*, *An. evansae* and *An. strodei*. Immature forms of *Anopheles triannulatus*, *Anopheles albitarsis* and *Anopheles rangeli* were also captured, but in small amounts. Larvae of *An. Pseudopunctipennis* fluctuated from late spring to autumn, when malaria cases occur in the area, whereas other anopheline larvae species fluctuated throughout the climatic seasons. An increase in the mean minimum temperature caused an increase in *An. Pseudopunctipennis* and *An. argyritarsis* abundance. Moreover, mean maximum temperature and water temperature greatly influenced the abundance of *An. pseudopunctipennis*, *An. evansae* and *An. strodei*. An increase of these variables resulted in an increase in their abundances. These climatic factors should be taken into account when implementing control measures of immature mosquito forms with the aim of reducing the number of larval habitats and larva production, which may ultimately result in the elimination of malaria in this area, (31).

To analyze whether *An. pseudopunctipennis* is a single population or a species complex in the country, morphometric variability was studied by conducting samplings not only in Argentina but also in Bolivia; in addition, a molecular study was performed considering only samples from Argentina.

A morphometric analysis was performed using a Discriminant Analysis. An "Unweighted Pair Group Method Analysis" (UPGMA) cluster analysis was performed to analyze the morphological similarity between populations, based on the Mahalanobis distances obtained in the discriminant analysis. The separation of Argentina and Bolivia populations was observed through characters associated with the length of the proboscis and palpomeres. Samples from Taruma (Santa Cruz) and Carrasco National Park (Cochabamba) in Bolivia appear together in the same clade. The polytomy observed in the cladistic analysis of Tucumán localities can be explained not only by the geographical proximity of El Molino and Iltico, but also by the fact that Molle Yaco stream, El Cadillal, Quebrada de Lules, Hornillo stream and La Sala are located in the transition area between the phytogeographic provinces of the Yungas and Chaco. Jujuy localities appear next to Potrero Las Tablas (Tucumán) in the same clade. All of Salta localities (Yungas) are together, and El Rey National Park appears closer to Aguas Blancas than to El Oculto. Again, all locations within the same clade belong to the same phytogeographic region, (32).

In the molecular study known as the demographic history and population structure of *Anopheles pseudopunctipennis* in Argentina based on the mitochondrial COI gene, 165 adult female *An. pseudopunctipennis* samples collected from 12 localities in three provinces of northwestern Argentina were analyzed. Demographic patterns suggest that *An. pseudopunctipennis* developed a single colonization process and that the ancestral haplotype is shared by all localities, as shown by several analyses, indicating a mitochondrial gene flow. Genetic differentiation was minimal and observed only from a locality between the northern and southern areas of the Yungas. The estimated population expansion time of this species was during the Holocene. These results suggest that regional control measures focused on the vector should be equally effective in both locations in the northern and southern areas of the Yungas, but also that genetic resistance to insecticides may rapidly disperse within this region, (33).

Since 2010 until today, studies within the framework of the National Malaria Program have been developed about the epidemiological aspects of malaria transmission in the rural area of the Argentine-Bolivian border, between Bermejo-Yacuiba (Bolivia) and Aguas Blancas-Salvador Mazza (Argentina).

One of the activities planned was the collection of specimens of *Anopheles* mosquitoes to detect the parasite that causes malaria, *Plasmodium vivax*. The selected sites included localities from both in Argentina and Bolivia, such as Yacuiba and Bermejo (Bolivia) and Acambuco and Salvador Mazza (Argentina).

Parasitological detection in mosquitoes was performed using molecular techniques. Of the total of 970 specimens of anopheles mosquitoes collected, *An. pseudopunctipennis* was the most abundant species, followed by *An. argyritarsis*, *An. strodei* and *An. evansae*. For *An. pseudopunctipennis*, all of the 34 pools analyzed were negative for *Plasmodium vivax*. Similarly, for *An. argyritarsis*, all of the 25 pools analyzed were negative for *P. vivax*.

No infection with *P. vivax* in anopheles mosquitoes was detected either considering the sampling sites or the periods in which the specimens were collected. In addition, no Anophels mosquitoes were found to be infected with *Plasmodium falciparum* or *Plasmodium malariae*, (34).

Contemporary entomological studies in northeastern Argentina (NEA)

As part of the malaria surveillance activities in Puerto Iguazú city, adult anopheles mosquitoes have been captured and immature forms (larvae and pupae) have been collected monthly since June 2012 to the present, in four localities of the province of Misiones with a history of malaria cases: Cabure-í, Puerto Iguazú, Puerto Libertad and Urugua-í, localities. In each locality, two CDC light traps with dry ice are placed, which remain active between 6 p.m. and 8 a.m.

In the same sites immature forms are collected from nearby ponds and streams using a 500-ml scoop, taking 20 scoops per larval habitat. Captured adults are transported to the laboratory inside their collection mesh, cooled in polypropylene boxes for counting and taxonomic identification. The immature forms are transported in labeled and duly refrigerated containers to the laboratory, where larvae are individually bred and pupae are massively bred until adults are obtained, (35).

In January 2014 anopheline capture using human bait was initiated in three of the four localities mentioned (Puerto Libertad, Puerto Iguazú and Urugua-í). For three consecutive days, between 6 p.m. and 00 a.m., two duly protected collectors using mechanical vacuum cleaners capture the Anopheles mosquitoes that land on them, during the first 50 minutes of every hour. The specimens caught are transferred to jars labeled with information on date and locality of capture.

In November 2013 a serological study was conducted using blood samples on filter paper to detect *Plasmodium* presence. Blood samples (n=380) were taken from residents from Puerto Iguazú(230 samples from Santa Rosa neighborhoods and 2000 hectáreas area) and Puerto Libertad (150 samples, from Bosetti, Itatí and Iprodha neighborhoods) by fingerstick in filter paper. DNA was extracted from blood samples on filter paper using two techniques: 1. a solution of cetyltrimethylammonium bromide homogenization (CTAB), and 2. Boiling technique (heat shock).

DNA amplification was performed using the technique of multiple semi-nested or conventional polymerase chain reaction (PCR), using generic primers. The sizes of the PCR products were estimated by 1.5% agarose gel electrophoresis. NF54 strain was used as a positive control (provided by the Malaria Group at the University of Antioquia, Medellin, Colombia) on filter paper. DNA was extracted from these controls by the two methods cited (CTAB and Boiling) to later obtain their dilutions.

The following results were obtained: to date, 427 specimens of Anopheles have been identified (356 with CDC traps and 71 with human bait) belonging to 13 species. The most abundant species was *An. evansae*, with 21.06%, followed by *An. benarrochi* (8.14%), *An. triannulatus* (4.77%), *An. mediopunctatus* (4.49%), *An. albitarsis* and *An. argyritarsis* (3.08%), *An. punctimacula* (2.52%), *An. strodei* (1.96%) and *An. deaneorum* (1.68%). The following species were present in less than 1%: *An. lutzii, An. fluminensis, An. galvaoi* (species that needs to be confirmed), *An. pinctipennis* and *An. parvus*. The species captured with human bait were: *An. albitarsis* (5.6%), *An. benarrochi* (14.08%), *An. evansae* (46.47%), *An. fluminensis* (4.22%), *An. strodei* (1.4%) and *An. triannulatus* (9.86%). In Puerto Iguazú the highest number of specimens with human bait was captured (54.92%), 39.43% in Urugua-í and only 4 specimens in Puerto Libertad. The greatest percentage of captures (91.54%) was recorded between 7 p.m. and 10 p.m. The analyses for *Plasmodium* detection were all negative.

Conclusion: To date the presence of *An. darlingi*, the only recognized vector of malaria in NEA, has not been detected in the study area, and the results of blood samples were negative for *Plasmodium*. These facts might put our country and that region close to the elimination phase of disease transmission. However, during recent outbreaks of Malaria no simultaneous mosquito samplings were performed and therefore it was not possible to accurately determine the species of anopheles acting as vectors. Considering that *An. argyritarsis, An. albitarsis, An. punctimacula, An.strodei* and *An. triannulatus*, detected during these studies, are considered vectors in other South American countries, it is necessary to continue with vector surveillance actions as well as epidemiological surveillance in the region.

The use of PCR is recommended as a screening method in epidemiological studies for the evaluation of National Malaria Control Programs, in studies aimed at early detection of parasitemia in treated patients who may have resistance to the antimalarials and as a reference test to evaluate new diagnostic methods, (M Stein Report, CNCV malaria consultant to the Ministry of Health, March 2015). During 2014, blood samples (a total of 639, with 273 being from males and 366 from females, of ages between 3 and 97 years) were taken to detect *Plasmodium*. Samplings were conducted in Puerto Iguazú (N=222), Comandante Andresito (N=57), Wanda (N=14) and Puerto Libertad (N=346), from March to June 2014. All the samples were processed using real time PCR technique for *Plasmodium* detection (positive control provided by Dr. Silvia Blair Trujillo and Malaria Group at the University of Antioquía, Medellín, Colombia). Of the processed samples, 86 were randomly selected using the controls provided by Honduras. All samples were negative for *Plasmodium*. So far no recent *P. vivax* or *falciparum* infection or recurrence of past *vivax* infections was detected in the study group, (ibid).

Evolution of Control

At this phase, evolution was heterogeneous and can be technically defined as of a "sustainable control", which basically consists of having the resources allocated in the most appropriate way and maintaining a level of activity that ensures a low transmission level or avoids transmission at all. In a country with multiple health priorities, the resources for a residual disease were variably assigned, because the available budget was shared with other vector-borne diseases such as dengue and Chagas, coexisting in the area. Particularly the former, since its reemergence in 1998, expresses with remarkable morbidity and annual recurrences, which makes coordinated approach to this type of pathologies complex.

Persistent malaria endemic area was smaller in relation to the previous descriptions of endemic distribution, with particular expression in the provinces of Salta, Jujuy, and

Tucumán in the northwest, and Missions in the northeast, both areas where the disease was endemic. Malaria epidemiological characteristics were:

- Seasonal variations in the occurrence of cases: in October, November and December and then from mid-February to March / April.
- Rural population is mostly affected.
- All age groups affected.
- Mild to moderate clinical expression and, except for cases of comorbidity, with outpatient treatment.
- *Plasmodium vivax* has been the only *Plasmodium* species present in all diagnosed cases in the endemic area in the last 20 years.
- The dominant vector is *Anopheles pseudopunctipennis*.

As previously mentioned, endemicity at this phase was maintained by the influence of migration flows in northwestern Argentina, on the Argentine-Bolivian border. This area in Salta province is a particularly complex site in the genesis of various epidemiological endemic problems such as the vector-borne diseases Dengue, Malaria, Chagas, which coexist and develop with a particular dynamics, especially with significant morbidity in the exposed population throughout the region.
Epidemiological experience in this region invariably shows that dengue and malaria epidemics in the country have been always directly related to situations of similar characteristics in Bolivia. The localities of Yacuiba and Bermejo have their corresponding mirror cities, Salvador Mazza and Aguas Blancas, and their influence areas overlap in all spheres of social life in the region, from ecological, climate, social, epidemiological points of views. Identifying the origin or location of patients is often impossible due to the proximity and similar lifestyles of both border populations. For all these reasons, vector-borne diseases in such a complex area must be dealt with using a combined approach to, at least, three diseases prevalent in the north: dengue, malaria and Chagas.

In the early 90s, an increasing trend of cases was observed on both sides of the Argentine-Bolivian border, reaching the highest numbers of the decade in 1996, as can be observed in Table 3.

Table N° 3. Cases of malaria until first ARBOL intervention in the border area.

Cases	1992	1993	1994	1995	1996
Cases in Argentina	643	758	948	1,055	2,076
Cases in Tarija	6,899	5,101	9,000	11,549	22,331

For that reason, health officials responsible for malaria activities in both countries decided to conduct the first joint intervention program under the ARBOL agreement. This agreement corresponds to the design of an approach strategy of diseases prevailing in the Argentine-Bolivian frontier area and was signed by both countries in the 90s. It was conducted in 1996, during the most important malaria epidemic occurred in the previous 20 years, with 2,076 cases reported on the Argentine side and 22,331 cases in Tarija department. The campaign lasted 45 days and involved 70 technicians (responsible for evaluation, spraying, sampling, workshops) and administrative workers (collection of information generated in the field). This operation consisted of the presence of Vector Control technical staff, 70 workers including field workers microscopists, administrators and supervisors, in the south in over 100 locations in Tarija department. These personnel traveled with the necessary resources (vehicles, fuel, insecticides and subsistence allowance) for conducting surveillance activities, residual house spraying, detection of patients with fever, sampling and administration of specific drugs. In short, a little more than 5,000 patients with malaria were detected, approximately 7,000 hematological samples were taken and more than 110 localities were systematically sprayed with residual insecticides.

For the operational activities, the staff was divided in two groups, each one working for about 22 days. The operations were developed in September and October, before the start of the rains in the area and when local anopheline population increases.

The period of activities was selected primarily for two reasons: on the one hand, in Argentina, the dynamics of malaria vector in the region includes a season of activity and reproduction of anopheles and, on the other hand, the rainy season starts in late October, which makes fieldwork very difficult.

After the first operative program, in 1996, the problem of dengue emerged; hence, successive operative activities were initially combined and, soon, Chagas also emerged, with the particular and serious ingredient of having a more complicated situation in Bolivia than in Argentina, which was related to the presence of vectors with high rates of resistance to pyrethroid insecticides as well as to control failure, (32). Then, from a practical point of view, it was possible to join efforts using the same methodology to approach the three prevalent vector-borne diseases. ARBOL operative activities were developed on a biannual or triennial basis using similar methods, with emphasis on spraying activity for treating Chagas, thereby ensuring cover for the other vectors involved. Malaria incidence decreased progressively at varying rates to 300 or 400 patients / year and even less in recent years.

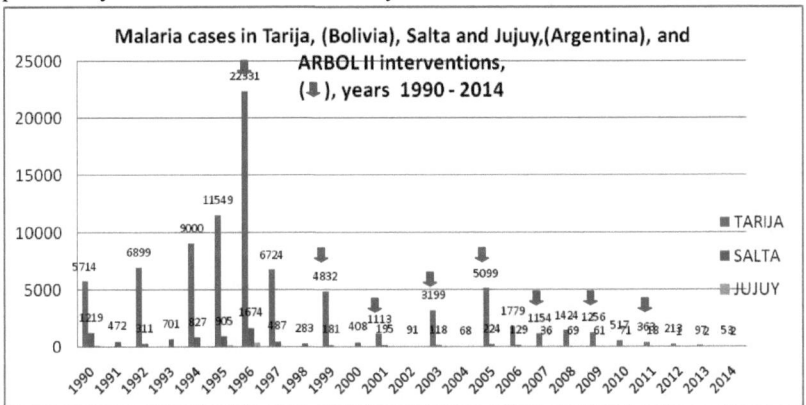

Fig. N° 13. Occurrence of malaria cases in Tarija department, Bolivia, and the provinces of Salta and Jujuy, Argentina, and ARBOL II interventions between 1990 and 2014, (PNP, Salta; SEDES, Tarija).

IPA por 1000 hab. 1990-2014 departamento de Tarija

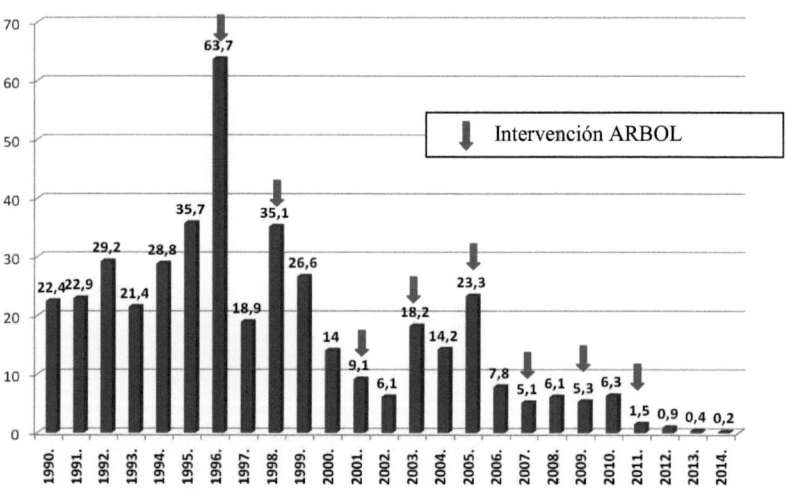

Figure N° 14 : Annual Parasite Index, (API), in Tarija department, 1990 – 2014 (Epidemiological week 40).
SEDES , Tarija

Table N° 4. Occurrence of malaria cases in Tarija department, Bolivia, and the
provinces of Salta, Jujuy, Tucuman, Corrientes and Misiones, Argentina,
between 1990 and 2014.

YEARS	TARIJA	SALTA	JUJUY	TUCUMAN	CORRIENTES	MISIONES
1990	5,714	1,219	194	26	0	88
1991	5,298	472	25	4	0	300
1992	6,899	311	62	0	1	259
1993	5,101	701	19	2	0	31
1994	9,000	827	98	4	1	5
1995	11,549	905	150	2	1	0
1996	22,331	1,674	358	3	8	0
1997	6,724	487	64	30	0	0
1998	5,746	283	31	3	1	5
1999	4,997	181	20	1	0	12
2000	4,832	408	27	1	0	1
2001	1,648	195	11	0	0	6
2002	1,113	91	1	0	0	31
2003	3,199	114	4	0	0	0
2004	2,497	106	8	0	0	0
2005	5,099	106	11	0	0	1
2006	1,779	129	15	0	0	65
2007	1,154	36	5	0	0	309
2008	1,424	80	0	0	0	19
2009	1,256	70	2	0	0	0
2010	1,517	56	0	0	0	0
2011	363	16	0	0	0	0
2012	213	14	1	0	0	0
2013	97	4	0	0	0	0
2014	53	4	0	0	0	0

Source: Sedes Tarija, Bolivia, and PNP, Argentina.

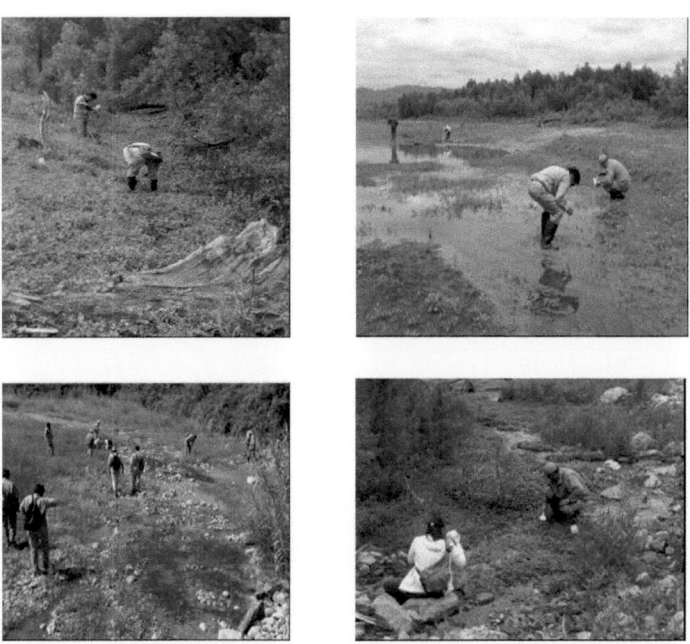

Photos N° 41, 42, 43, 44. Technicians in search of immature stages in streams near Itiyuro dam, Aguaray, Salta.

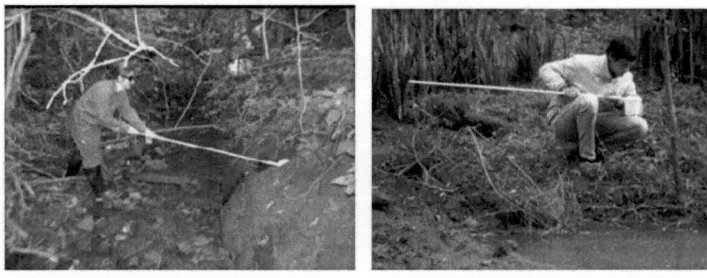

Photos N° 45 and 46. Team members in search of immature stages in streams in a settlement of Puerto Iguazú municipality, Misiones.

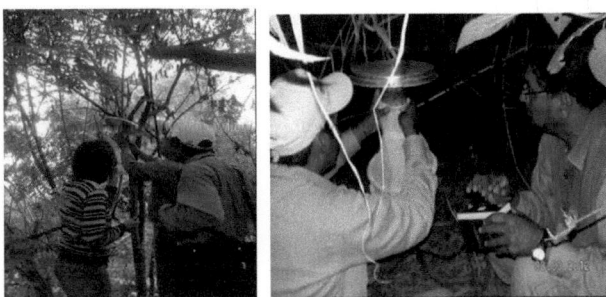

Photos Nº 47 and 48. Placement of an entomological trap in the periurban area of Salta city, and Orán settlement.

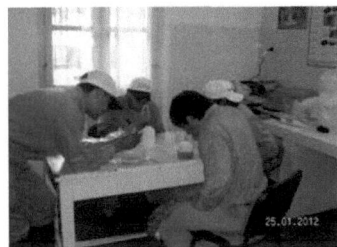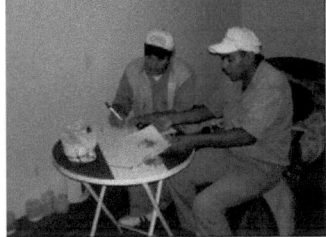

Photos Nº 49 and 50. Entomological material in the laboratory; classification process.

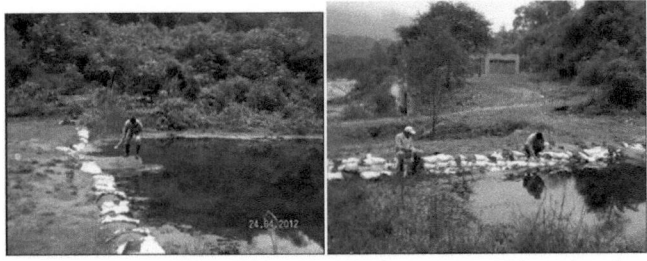

Photos Nº 51 and 52. Technicians in search of immature stages in streams near Itiyuro dam, Aguaray, Salta.

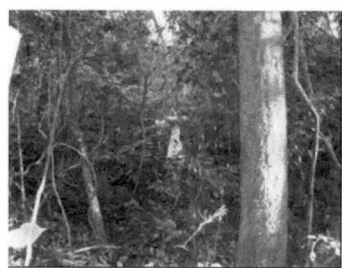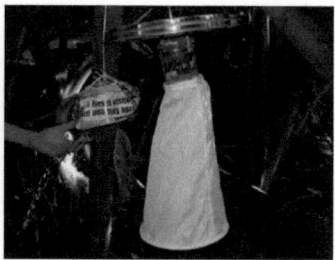

Photo No. 53 and 54. Placement of an entomological trap in Acambuco area.

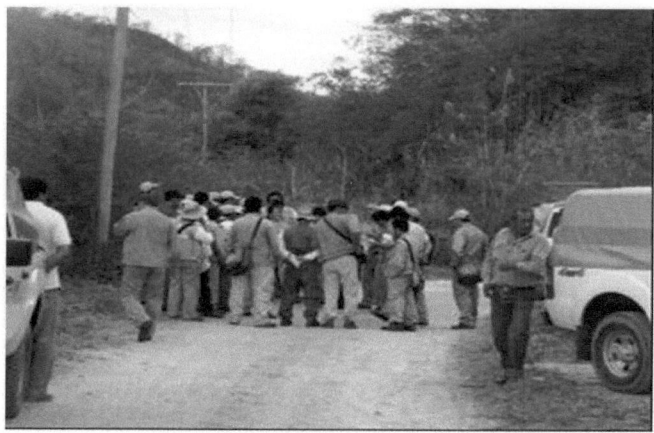

Photo No 55. Meeting in the field to coordinate actions.

All of the operative activities are linked through a series of related activities based on the proposal for elimination of autochthonous malaria transmission, such as conducting operational research activities, locating potential and actual sources of anopheles breeding sites through geo-referencing, adjusting adult anopheles traps with locally developed technology and controlled testing of products for prevention and vector control.

FOURTH PHASE
2009-2015

At the end of the previous phase, in 2008, given the epidemiological evolution of the endemic disease in the country, it was possible to define epidemiological criteria for stratifying risk areas. Thus, two areas were defined: area or stratum 1 and 2. Area 1 had low epidemiological risk, but the highest risk in the country; here, no epidemics occur, the annual parasite index is $0.01\%_0$ and the occurrence of cases is occasional. Area or stratum 2 has a similar parasite index, no autochthonous cases occur, and includes the exclusive surveillance area, (22).

From the operative standpoint, this meant the allocation of activities with a differential criterion. Area one covers Oran and San Martin departments in Salta province and comprises about 4000 homes in scattered rural areas, with more than half of them being of difficult access. Here, surveillance activities are conducted, comprising entomological evaluation, detection of patients with fever, blood sampling from asymptomatic patients living in the risk area, and annual application of pyrethroid insecticides, particularly in the months considered of greatest entomological risk, from September to December.

Area two, of exclusive surveillance, where no autochthonous cases have occurred for at least seven years, and that comprises the ramal area of Jujuy, El Carmen, Palpalá, General Belgrano, San Pedro and Ledesma departments in Jujuy province, Anta department in Salta province and Puerto Iguazú municipality in Misiones province. In this area, monitoring activities comprise the visit to health centers and laboratories of volunteers to get information about any febrile cases that may arise. In the area, entomological surveys that tend to characterize the peculiarities of the local fauna are also periodically performed, (see M Stein's report).

Since 2008, between 200 and 300 cases a year were recorded, with interannual variations; approximately between 50% and 70% of cases are imported from abroad, with a gradual slow decreasing trend, reaching 72 imported cases in 2010, and no autochthonous cases.

Since 2010, the National Malaria Program (PNP), under the National Ministry of Health, develops intensified control and surveillance activities in order to maintain the elimination of malaria autochthonous transmission in the endemic area.

THE PATH TO CERTIFICATION OF ELIMINATION

For over a decade Argentina has had an annual parasite index of less than 1%$_o$, with no records of autochthonous cases for five years now. With these basic summary indicators, Argentina can submit a request to the World Health Organization for locally transmitted malaria elimination certification. For this, and at the organization request, the National Malaria Program has elaborated a series of documents that illustrate and describe the epidemiological dynamics of malaria in Argentina in the last 10 years, as well as supporting documentation, including the following items:

1. Action plan for preventing malaria reintroduction.
2. Organizational structure of the malaria department's activities regarding general health services, with detailed budgets and staff information.
3. Annual malaria surveillance reports covering the past 10 years.
4. Complete information on the malaria active foci for five years preceding the last autochthonous case, with supporting maps.
5. A National Registry of malaria cases with individual case investigation forms on all malaria infections detected in the country for the past three years
6. Reports of quality-assurance activities for diagnosis
7. Recent antimalarial drugs policy.
8. Detailed entomological and vector control activities.
9. Reports provided by independent committees about malaria, surveillance system, entomological activities and vector control.
10. Recent published and unpublished research reports about malaria epidemiology and vectors.
11. Legislation / regulations related to malaria and vector control.
12. Intersectoral collaboration reports.

13. Inter-country reports about coordination mechanisms in the border area, wherever relevant

ACTION PLAN FOR THE PREVENTION OF MALARIA REINTRODUCTION
Stratum ONE, Salta (Oran and San Martin departments)

The risk area of these departments includes:

1. A group of localities north of Aguas Blancas (Orán), on the east bank of Tarija River, on the Argentine-Bolivian border.
2. Another risk area covering Aguaray rural area, San Martin department, and nearby localities.
3. The sanitary sectors of Salvador Mazza municipality, some of which are rural and periurban, bordering with the Bolivian localities of San José de Pocitos and Yacuiba.

Localities / Sites	Orán Department	
	Number of houses	Number of inhabitants
Aguas Blancas	125	625
Porcelana	15	60
Aujoncito	12	50
Media Luna	5	20
Pozo el Mate	5	20
Algarrobito	18	70
Volcán	18	70
Volcán Trasfondo	5	15
San Telmo	6	25
Trasfondo San Telmo	5	15
Trementinal	18	70
Isla de los Novillos	5	20
Corredero	4	15
Astillero	9	35
Madrejones	18	70

Cañaveral	3	10
	271	1,190
San Martín Department		
Colodro – Aguaray	11	45
Macueta bajo – Aguaray	30	125
Campo Largo - Aguaray	45	180
Acambuco – Aguaray	150	630
	158	980
San Martín Department		
	Number of houses	**Number of inhabitants**
Capiazuti	100	583
Campo Durán	136	799
Agua blanca	45	270
Campo blanco	52	312
La Angostura	12	72
Algarrobal	3	12
Tobantirenda	102	606
Caraparí	150	864
Dique Itiyuro	30	174
Arenales	150	878
San Antonio	12	48
Madrejones	7	36
Playa ancha	12	68
Yerba buena	109	651
La bendición	24	135
Monte Sinaí	18	106
El Obraje (x)	27	165
San Cayetano (x)	27	159
La Pista (x)	177	1,108
Villa Las Rosas	35	201
Justo Juez	100	578

Ba. Ferroviario	491	1,964
Ba Belgrano	23	138
La Playa (x)	109	642
Sector Cinco (x)	128	755
San Martín (x)	232	755
La Toma (x)	18	928
El Chorro (x)	182	98
El Sauzal (x)	168	1,103
Total	2,679	14,446

(x): Adjacent to border area

A surveillance system was established in the mentioned area. Technicians traveled throughout the risk area once a month, visiting approximately 4,000 homes, and taking blood samples of at least 10% of the assisted population.

Contacts with the primary health care network services were intensified; interaction with health workers in the area occurs during each biweekly visit. Nonspecific febrile syndromes that are not confirmed as malaria cases are derived to local health centers and / or regional hospitals.

In 2012 and 2013 updating meetings of doctors, biochemists and nurses have addressed the differential diagnosis of acute febrile syndrome with emphasis on regional pathologies including malaria.

Workshops about malaria microscopy were conducted for technicians and biochemists, in Metán, Orán, Salta and Tartagal.

Updating workshops about malaria surveillance for national, local and NGOs technicians were conducted in Salta, Tartagal and Puerto Iguazú.

Sanitary entomology workshops with emphasis on malaria vectors, distribution, taxonomy, bionomics of prevalent vectors: Salta, Tartagal, Puerto Iguazú with participation of national, provincial, municipal and NGO technicians.

Training Activities (2012 – 2013)

Activity	Topics	Participants	Provenance
Workshop	Differential diagnosis of acute febrile syndrome with emphasis on regional pathology	Medical doctors, biochemists, nurses	Salta city, and localities from Salta province
Conferences	Zoonosis Development of issues related to malaria clinics, diagnosis, treatment and epidemiology	Medical doctors, biochemists, nurses, health workers	Salta, and localities of the province
Workshop	Malaria epidemiological surveillance. Low-transmission areas	Field technicians from the national government	Salta, Orán, Tartagal, Güemes, R. de la Frontera, S. Mazza, Puerto Iguazú
Workshop	Malaria microscopic diagnosis	Technicians, biochemists	Salta, Orán, Tartagal, Metán, Puerto Iguazú
Workshop	Malaria entomological aspects: vectors, distribution, bionomics, taxonomy of prevalent species	Technicians from the national and local governments	Salta, Orán, Tartagal, Puerto Iguazú

Stratum TWO

Stratum TWO is the area with only surveillance activities and without insecticide spraying. This stratum comprises the areas with no cases reported in recent years and with no autochthonous cases for at least three years. It includes the ramal region in Jujuy province, with El Carmen, Santa Barbara, Palpalá, San Pedro, Ledesma and General Belgrano departments, a 13,143 km² area and a population of approximately 575,700 residents; Anta department in Salta, a 21,945 km² area and 57,411 residents; and Iguazu city in Misiones province, 625 km² and 82,227 residents (PNP technical report 2011).

Misiones (locality of Puerto Iguazú)

The last outbreak in the area occurred in 2007 in Puerto Iguazú and produced 309 cases, particularly in the areas of Puerto Libertad, 2000 hectáreas area, and Santa Rosa neighborhood.

The primary health care service in the area has clinical specialties and a basic laboratory for diagnostic testing of cases referred by the health team and health volunteers. The health team detects patients with acute febrile syndrome in health centers and hospitals and is able to treat common cases (passive search).

Once a month a PNP technician team visits the risk area (defined as a residual inactive area), and conduct house-to-house surveillance, taking blood samples from approximately 10% of asymptomatic patients.

Clinical update workshops about febrile syndromes with emphasis on regional pathology, including malaria diagnosis, have been conducted for doctors and biochemists. Likewise, training workshops in malaria epidemiological surveillance were conducted for national, provincial, and municipal vector technicians as well as those belonging to the Mundo Sano Foundation from Puerto Iguazú.

From the entomological point of view, samplings are conducted at four sites in the risk area (Puerto Iguazú municipality), to characterize the local anopheline fauna. Two trials with human bait have been performed, and four similar tests in the risk area are planned to be held.

The technicians responsible for the sanitary sector are in permanent contact with the provincial health system, particularly with the system of Primary Health Care, with emphasis on detection of fever cases and with the laboratory area in order to record diagnosed fever cases.

In summary:
- Stratum ONE (Endemic) 28,149 km² and 250,000 residents
- Stratum TWO: (Surveillance) 35,213 km² and 907,297 residents

According to the definition of the World Health Organization, Argentina has technically achieved the status of elimination of autochthonous transmission of malaria. Therefore, it is possible to address the reintroduction prevention stage in the country based on the following considerations:

1. No autochthonous cases were recorded in the endemic area in the last four years
2. A surveillance system has been established in the risk area.
3. Health service providers have been have been trained in the field for the detection and identification of fever cases suspected of malaria.
4. There is an organizational structure suited for factual possibilities of the program.

EPILOGUE

Long has been the path for generations of Argentines, seeking to mitigate or avoid the evils of malaria. Even in adverse circumstances, with many difficulties, with the inevitable setbacks of a complicated and difficult process that does not end. As it did not end in those countries they amounted to certify the elimination of autochthonous malaria, and still pass the long transition of the Prevention of reintroduction of cases. So many lives had the disease and its consequences, as so many lives were given to the fight against this disease. These pages have been written as a modest tribute to all those who lived an authentic epic ....

THANKS TO:

- My family that is accompanying me;
- Co-workers who are active in the provinces of the endemic area;
- Heads of sectors, Carlos Vega, Misiones; Jorge Kuruc (Corrientes); Hector Janútolo (Tartagal); Bernardo Carrazán (Oran); Juan Leaño (Ledesma); Aldo Cocha (San Pedro de Jujuy); Hugo Landriel, San S. de Jujuy); Benito Quiquinto (Rosario de la Frontera), employees committed to their function;
- New generations of technicians in the national malaria program, hoping continuity of task;
- Maria Julia Dantur entomologist consultant National Malaria Program, NOA area, tireless researcher and source of encouragement to our technicians. .
- Maria Concepcion Montero, Biochemistry, consultant National Malaria Program, NOA area; specialist diagnosis of malaria.
- Marina Stein, entomologist, consultant of the national malaria program, NEA area, committed collaborator in her work area;
- Carlos Ripoll, an epidemiologist at the Ministry of Public Health of the province of Jujuy;
- Hector Masuh, chemical, pesticide management expert, CIPEIN, Buenos Aires;
- Health Ministry Officials that have accompanied the task over the years;

BIBLIOGRAPHY

1. Eliseo Cantón. El paludismo y su Geografía en la República Argentina. Buenos Aires. Imprenta La Universidad, 1891.

2. Antenor Alvarez. Paludismo. El saneamiento de la ciudad de Santiago del Estero. Memoria presentada a la Primera Conferencia Panamericana de la Cruz Roja. Doctor Antenor Alvarez. Buenos Aires, 379901-Talleres S.A. Casa Peuser, 1923.

3. Delfino JC, An. Dep. Nac. Hig. IX-435-1902. Rev. Soc. Méd.Arg.X - 435-1902.

4. Guillermo Paterson C. Las fiebres palúdicas en Jujuy. Anales del Departamento Nacional de Higiene. 18(1911):31-57.

5. Mirta Fleitas. Epidemias y endemias en Jujuy durante la década de 1930. Mirta Fleitas. KAIROS. Revista de Temas Sociales. ISSN 1514-9331.Publicación de la Universidad Nacional de San Luis. Proyecto Culturas Juveniles Urbanas Año 10. N° 18 Noviembre de 2006.

6. Alfredo Kohn Loncarica, Abel Agüero y Norma Isabel Sánchez, Nacionalismo e Internacionalismo en las ciencias de la salud: el caso de la lucha antipalúdica en la Argentina(3) *Asclepio-Vol* XLIX-2-1997, Asclepio, Vol 49, No 2 (1997).

7. Ley 5195 Sobre el Paludismo. Decreto Reglamentario. Ministerio del Interior. Buenos Aires. Imprenta y Encuadernación de la Policía, 1911.

8. Muhlens P, Dios R, Petrocchi J y Zuccarini A. En Estudios sobre Paludismo y Hematología en el Norte Argentino por los Doctores Pedro Muhlens, Roberto L Dios, Juana Petrocchi, y Señor Juan Zuccarini. Revista del Instituto bacteriológico del DNH 4, No. 3, (1925) del DNH.

9. Barbieri, A. La cuestión paludismo. Su profilaxis en Argentina. Conferencia Sanitaria Nacional, pp 1-14; Departamento Nacional de Higiene, 1923, Buenos Aires.

10. Barbieri Antonio. El problema de saneamiento antimalárico en la Argentina. Consideraciones y antecedentes. Anales del Departamento Nacional de Higiene, 25, No. 2 (1919): 21-37.

11. Shannon RC; Davis NC y E. del Ponte. La distribución del *Anopheles pseudopunctipennis* y su relación con el paludismo en la Argentina. Revista del Instituto del DNH, 4, No. 7 (1927):679-705, Buenos Aires.

12. Alvarado Carlos A. Métodos de lucha antipalúdica en la República Argentina. Informe presentado a la Décima conferencia Sanitaria Panamericana por el Dr. Miguel Sussini, presidente del DNH. Boletín Sanitario del DNH 3 (1938), 891-904.

13. Bachman Alois. Programa de lucha para llevarse a cabo en Famaillá contra los anófeles y sus larvas. Anales del DNH. 27, No. 3, (1921):117-37.

14. Eric D. Carter. Enemy in the blood. Malaria, Environment, and Development in Argentina. The University of Alabama Press, 2012, Tuscaloosa, Alabama 35487-0380.

15. Sierra e Iglesias Jobino Pedro. Carlos Alberto Alvarado. Vida y Obra. Comisión Bicameral examinadora de Obras de autores salteños., Salta 1993.

16. Zaidenberg Mario. Paludismo en Argentina. En Actualizaciones en Artropodología Sanitaria Argentina. Serie de enfermedades transmisibles, pp 283-289. Publicación monográfica, Red Argentina de Estudio de Artrópodos Vectores de Enfermedades Humanas, noviembre de 2002.

17. Siquot JC y Silvetti Peña L. Planteamiento actual de la lucha antipalúdica en la República Argentina, pp 377-380. En Primeras Jornadas Entomoepidemiológicas argentinas, Primera parte, Buenos Aires, República Argentina, 1959.

18. Alvarez A. Un enemigo menos?: Erradicación y reemergencia del paludismo en la Argentina, 1940-1960. Diálogos Revista Electrónica de Historia ISSN 1409- 469 X. Número especial 2008. Dirección web: http://historia.fcs.ucr.ac.cr/dialogos.htm

19. Alvarado, CA. "Control de las Enfermedades Transmitidas por Mosquitos". Revista Mensual de Oficina Sanitaria Panamericana (Washington) 27, n° 12, (Diciembre 1948): 1105-182.

20. Bejarano JFR. Anopheles de la República Argentina y sus relaciones con el Paludismo. Primeras Jornadas entomoepidemiológicas Argentinas, Primera parte, 1959; pp 305-329. Buenos Aires, República Argentina.

21. Alvarado CA, Ousset JH, Roffe J, Umana AC y Heredia R; 1951, Notas sobre Epidemiología del Paludismo del Litoral. 1ª. Reunión Pan. Enf de Chagas. Tucumán, julio 1949, fsc. 3, pág. 23, Tucumán.

22. Lifshitz J, Umana CA, Vergara JJ y Heredia RL: 1946 Anal Inst. Med Reg. (Univ Nac de Tucumán, 1-349.

23. Zaidenberg M. Control of Malaria in Argentina Part II. Rev Arg Zoon and Enf emerg. Vol. IX, No. 1, pp 6 - 10, April 2014.

24. Referencia geográfica del límite norte de argentina...

25. Dantur MJ; Zaidenberg M; Almirón W. Fluctuación estacional *An pseudopunctipennis* (DIPTERA: CULICIDAE) en un área palúdica de Salta,

Argentina. Entomol. Vect. 10 (4): 457- 468,2003. ISSN 0328-0381. Universidade Gama Filho.

26. Dantur MJ; Zaidenberg M; Almirón W. Distribución espacial de *An pseudopunctipennis* en la Yungas de Salta, Argentina. Rev Saúde Pública, 2005, 39, (4), 565-70.

27. Satellite-derived NDVI, LST, and climate factors driving the distribution and abundance of *Anopheles* mosquitoes in a former malarious area in northwest Argentina,(Pages 36-45). María Julia Dantur Juri, Elizabet Estallo, Walter Almirón, Mirta Santana, Paolo Sartor, Mario Lamfri and Mario Zaidenberg. J Vector Ecology, 2015. http://onlinelibrary.wiley.com/doi/10.1111/jvec.12130/abstract

28. Abundance patterns of *Anopheles pseudopunctipennis* and *Anopheles argyritarsis* in northwestern Argentina MJ Dantur; G Claps; M Santana; M Zaidenberg. Acta Tropica 115, (2010), 234-241.

29. Malaria journal in two localities in north-western Argentina. Dantur MJ; Zaidenberg M; Claps G; W Almirón. Malaria Journal 2009, 818.

30. Longitudinal study of the species composition and spatio-temporal abundance of Anopheles larvae in a malaria risk area in Argentina. Dantur, MJ; Galante G; Zaidenberg M; Almirón W; Claps, G and M Santana. Memórias do Instituto Oswaldo Cruz. ID is MIOC-2013-0186.

31. Morphometric variability of *Anopheles pseudopunctipennis* (DIPTERA: CULICIDAE) from different ecoregions of Argentina and Bolivia. María J Dantur Juri, Jonathan Liris, Juan C Navarro, Roberto Rodriguez and Gary N Fritz. Florida Entomologist 94(3) September 2011.

32. Dantur Juri MJ, Moreno M, Mónica J Prado Izaguirre MJ, Navarro JC , Zaidenberg MO, Almirón WR, Claps GL and Conn JE. Historia demográfica y estructura poblacional de *Anopheles pseudopunctipennis* en Argentina basado en el gen mitocondrial COI. Parasites & Vectors 2014, 7:423. http://www. parasiteandvectors.com/content/7/1/423.

33. Anales Alberto Roemmers. M. J. Dantur Juri; M. Zaidenberg; M. Abril; C. Veggiani Aybar; G. Galante; M. S. Olea; E. Laci; C. Laci; D. Carrizo; A. Alancay; J. Romero; V. González; A. De Lucio; P. Mula Lozano; P. Berzosa Díaz. Epidemiología de la malaria en el Noroeste de Argentina: dinámica de la transmisión. Anales Fundación Roemmers, años 2010 – 2012, pp 145-157.

34. Zaidenberg, M. Evolución entomológica del Municipio de Salvador Mazza, departamento San Martín, Provincia de Salta, Argentina, 1998 – 2004. XIIIa. Reunión Intergubernamental INCOSUR/Chagas, Bs.As., Argentina, Marzo de 2004. OPS/DPC/CD/308/04 Original: Español.

ANNEX

- **Organizational structure of the National Malaria Program**

The National Malaria Program (PNP) has provided field service for over 70 years; in the beginning, its territorial distribution included more than 250,000 km^2 and involved eight northern and central provinces.

In recent years, after about 30 years of activities involving sustainable control, the active endemic area has been reduced to San Martin and Orán departments in Salta province, 28,000 km^2, and surveillance Ramal area, south of Salta province, and Puerto Iguazú in Misiones.

The National Malaria Program is based in the capital city of Salta, with a technical and an administrative area. The technical area has a Field Operations Department in charge of planning activities for prevention and control of malaria, dengue, Chagas and Leishmaniasis. A number of additional offices include Statistics Department, Malaria Referral Laboratory for all samples collected in the field, material storage, insecticides, spraying machines, vehicle area, administration, treasury, maintenance and reception area. Thirty-seven people work in Salta, including professionals, technicians and administrative workers.

Other bases that depend on Salta operating base include the following: Tartagal, Orán, Salvador Mazza, General Güemes, Rosario de la Frontera, in Salta province; San Pedro, Ledesma and San Salvador de Jujuy in Jujuy province; each base is ran by a Head of Sector and personnel with respective assigned function.

Puerto Libertad and Puerto Iguazú, in Misiones province, are bases that until 10 years ago belonged administratively to the Salta base; today they can be regarded as operational bases that support Malaria surveillance activities in the province of Misiones.

Each of these bases has a variable number of mainly technical and administrative personnel. The Orán, Tartagal, Ledesma and San Pedro bases have a laboratory for malaria diagnosis.

AVAILABLE RESOURCES, 2014

BASE	Human Resources	Vehicles	Heavy machinery	Portable equipment	Lab
Salta	37	12	4	22	Yes
Orán	27	8	3	23	Yes
Tartagal	16	5	2	21	Yes
G. Güemes	1	1	0	2	0
R. de la Frontera	5	2	0	5	0
San Pedro	5	3	0	6	Yes
Ledesma	7	3	1	6	Yes
S.S. de Jujuy	5	3	0	5	Yes
S. Mazza	3	1	0	3	Yes
Puerto Iguazú	10	4	3	13	Yes (MSPM)
Corrientes	13	7	3	13 ULV 13 Resid	Yes (MSPC)
TOTAL	124	44	16		

MPHM: Ministry of Public Health of Misiones
MPHC: Ministry of Public Health of Corrientes

PNP has a stable budget for resource allocation including:

ANNUAL BUDGET ALLOCATION, PNP,
YEARS 2010, 2011, 2012, 2013, 2014

Human resources and technical assistance	851,000
Training /Education	89,000
Insecticide and spraying materials	50,000
Diagnosis	15,000
Anti-malarial drugs	30,000
Input purchase and management	10,700
Communication and dissemination of preventive actions	12,000
Monitoring and evaluation	25,000
Total (Argentine pesos)	1,082,700

- **Annual surveillance records of the last 10 years.**

PNP has notification records of cases from the last 15 years.

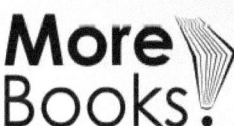
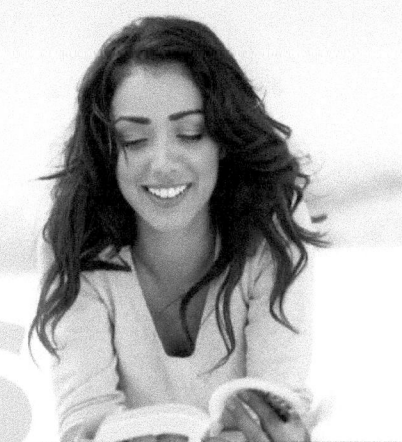

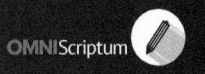

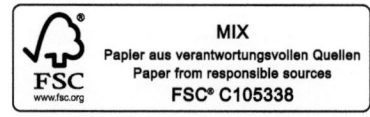

Printed by Books on Demand GmbH, Norderstedt / Germany